52-WEEK DEVOTIONAL
for
GIRLS

PRAYERS FOR GROWTH AND INSPIRATION

JASEÑA S'VANI

Illustrations by
Clairice Gifford

ROCKRIDGE
PRESS

For general information on our other products and services or to obtain technical support, please contact our Customer Care Department within the United States at (866) 744-2665, or outside the United States at (510) 253-0500.

Rockridge Press publishes its books in a variety of electronic and print formats. Some content that appears in print may not be available in electronic books, and vice versa.

Scripture quotations marked (GNT) are from the Good News Translation in Today's English Version, Second Edition, Copyright © 1992 by American Bible Society. Used by Permission.

Scripture quotations marked (HCSB) are taken from the Holman Christian Standard Bible®, Copyright © 1999, 2000, 2002, 2003, 2009 by Holman Bible Publishers. Used by permission. Holman Christian Standard Bible®, Holman CSB®, and HCSB® are federally registered trademarks of Holman Bible Publishers.

Scripture quotations marked (ICB) are quoted from the International Children's Bible®, Copyright ©1986, 1988, 1999, 2015 by Tommy Nelson. Used by permission.

Scripture quotations marked (NKJV) are taken from the New King James Version®. Copyright © 1982 by Thomas Nelson. Used by permission. All rights reserved.

Scripture quotations marked (NIV) are taken from the Holy Bible, New International Version®, NIV®. Copyright © 1973, 1978, 1984, 2011 by Biblica, Inc.® Used by permission of Zondervan. All rights reserved worldwide. www.zondervan.com. The "NIV" and "New International Version" are trademarks registered in the United States Patent and Trademark Office by Biblica, Inc.®

Interior and Cover Designer: Linda Snorina
Art Producer: Samantha Ulban
Editor: Laura Bryn Sisson
Production Manager: Holly Haydash
Production Editor: Melissa Edeburn

Illustrations © Clairice Gifford.
Author photo courtesy of Divine Photography.

ISBN: Print 978-1-64876-364-9
eBook 978-1-64876-365-6

R0

A toda mi familia...los quiero mucho.

Introduction

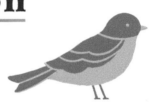

Dear girls,

When I was your age, I appeared to have everything going for me. My parents were together and successful. I was a strong athlete, and I got along with pretty much everyone. But no one knew that I was facing challenges. I struggled to know my true worth and to find good relationships. Maybe you can relate!

Why did my challenges never break me? During my entire life, God has been my silver lining. Even when I didn't know who He really was, He was there to protect me and help me feel whole.

Yes, I have experienced some pain and been knocked off my feet, thinking I would never make it. I've made some bad decisions. I've hurt friends, disappointed my parents, and disappointed myself. But then I chose God. In some of my lowest times, I heard the quiet whisper of God telling me, "I still love you. I will never leave you." God has shown me that, no matter what happens, He has the final say and He always keeps his promises!

Even when things seem really hard, this book will remind you that God always has your back. The reflections in this book might challenge the way you think about things. You might find that you're inspired to have deep, personal conversations with your friends and family members about how you're feeling and about your relationship with God. Rethinking perspectives is sometimes scary, exciting, or both! But God will be right there with you, helping you grow.

There are 52 entries in this book—one for each week of the year. You don't have to follow them in any particular order. Each is designed to be reflected on for the entire week.

Together we'll explore some of the everyday ups and downs, from friendships to school. No matter what you're facing each week, God is with you and will help you do your best!

Biblical Writings

The Bible is a collection of many individuals' writings, in many languages, about Jesus's life and his ministry thousands of years ago. The Bible's many translations have allowed people all over the world to read and learn about Jesus. Throughout this book, you'll encounter different translations, and if you decide to read the Bible, you might find another translation that you like.

If you have your own Bible, awesome! If you don't, it's easy to gain access to scripture. Resources like BibleHub.com and BibleGateway.com allow you to read the entire Bible on your computer or smartphone. You can also use one of my personal favorites, The Bible App by YouVersion.

In the Bible, you'll encounter narratives, psalms, and letters. Narratives are stories about what someone encountered, psalms are songs of praise, and I'm pretty sure you already know what a letter is. In this book, you'll find all these forms of writing. Let's dive in.

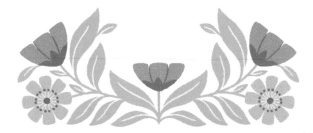

I'm stressing out—I need some space!

Do you ever feel really drained or just frazzled? Maybe you have a tough math test this week, your siblings are totally annoying while you're trying to study, and you had a tiff with your bestie. Then to top off all the drama, you still have to do your daily house chores and other homework. It can be a bit overwhelming, right?

This is where boundaries come to the rescue! You might think boundaries are about blocking negative people out of your life or maybe even not befriending someone who doesn't like the same things as you do. Those are boundaries, sure, but it's even bigger than that!

The point of setting healthy boundaries is to make sure you have a safe place to look inward and reflect. It's like putting a protective bubble around your spirit so you can protect your peace and energy. Boundaries allow you to accept that you are only so strong and need time to rest. It's okay to draw an invisible line around your personal space when you need a rest from a fast-paced world.

The best place you can learn about setting boundaries is by looking at how Jesus lived. He constantly took time alone to pray and be in solitude with God (see Matthew 14:23 and Mark 1:35). By having these boundaries for himself He could "recharge" and focus on the most important thing—spending time with God.

When you pray, go into your room, and when you have shut your door, pray to your Father who is in the secret place; and your Father who sees in secret will reward you openly.

Matthew 6:6 NKJV

Reflect

Figure out a space in or around your home where you can be alone. When life overwhelms, you have your own "secret" space for praying—maybe under a staircase, a spot near the backyard garden, or even a corner of your bedroom or closet.

Respond

Sit in your private space and ponder: "How can I set some positive boundaries in my world?" Maybe you can ditch some extracurricular activities or set your bedtime a bit earlier to read or pray before you doze off. Jot down your ideas here:

_____

_____

_____

> God, boundaries are hard! I don't want to hurt anyone's feelings by telling them no. Can you help me understand how to set good boundaries?

Ugh! I'm not being treated with kindness.

Bullying can be about name-calling in a school hallway or even getting punched on the playground. These obviously are not ideal scenarios, but in today's world, bullying also has another arena—the Internet. It has no preference and, unfortunately, anyone can experience it.

When I was in high school, I was bullied by a group of three girls. I remember feeling angry, insecure, and sad to the point that I didn't even want to go to school just so I could avoid them. I didn't know what to do at first because I felt embarrassed, but with the support of my parents, I found the courage to speak with my principal and teachers about what was going on. If you feel similarly to how I did, be encouraged to stand tall and confident. Lean on a trusted adult to help you navigate your situation and, most importantly, don't forget that you are *loved*.

The reality about bullies is that they are actually the ones who are most insecure about themselves. Ironic, right? Bullies are typically the people who are the loudest and most obnoxious on the outside . . . and are the ones who are truly suffering the most on the inside. Even though they might appear to be confident in who they are, it could actually be the complete opposite—they don't believe in themselves! Oftentimes, bullies will try to push other people down in hopes that it will make them feel better about themselves. Doesn't make sense at all, does it?

So what should you do if you or someone you know is getting bullied? First, you should remember that even though bullies are downright mean, they are still human just like you. All they want are reactions out of their victims because they want attention. While your knee-jerk reaction might be to treat them unkindly right back, try embracing a new perspective—one of love! Stand firm in who you are: someone who is strong, empathetic, joyful, and loving. When it comes down to it, sometimes bullies just need a true friend, and that could be you.

If you have a sneaking feeling that you yourself might not be treating people with kindness, I want you to take a moment to pause, think, and ask yourself a few questions:

"Why am I being mean to other girls?"

"How am I benefiting from hurting other people who are just like me?"

"Am I running from something deeper?"

Oftentimes, we might not realize that our behaviors are really just reflections of what we might be dealing with inside. Instead of projecting those emotions onto others, try to spend some time processing what it is you're really struggling with on the inside. It's only then that you will be able to find peace and shift your actions to make better choices.

Whether you're struggling with the urge to treat people unkindly, or you're seeing unkindness around you, trust in God to guide you to choose love.

Forget about the wrong things people do to you. You must not try to get even. Love your neighbor as you love yourself. I am the Lord.

Leviticus 19:18 ICB

Reflect

If you're feeling bullied by someone, repeat the following statement to yourself. Um, wait . . . back that up! Say this even if you *don't* know a bully: "I stand in the truth that I'm loved by God. Nothing anyone thinks about me can change that!"

Respond

Break out your Bible! Read Psalm 121 with a friend or by yourself. Write down a list of ways that God watches over you and gives you strength. Know that God is with you . . .

_____

_____

_____

_____

_____

_____

Lord, I know you love me, and I know it makes you sad to see your children in pain. Will you give me the strength to stand firm on your truth that you love me no matter what? Amen.

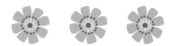

I'm having trouble staying positive.

No matter what happens in your day-to-day life, there is always *a lot* to be grateful for. There might be times when you get a bad grade or turn your nose up at lunch, but don't you feel happier when you remember how blessed you are to be getting an education and complete meals? If you always strive to have a positive outlook, you'll find many pockets of joy.

Say, for example, you've been relentlessly griping to your parents about your allowance or being allowed to stay up later at night. Stop that right now, and try a little experiment. Instead of the hissy fits, step into a happy place. Have fun spending your allowance on a new item, like stickers or a lip balm. And be joyful spending your bedtime doing something you love, such as writing in your journal or quietly meditating.

The great news is that joy is a choice. Even in unpleasant situations, you get to decide how you'll respond. Shift your perspective and make a pinkie-promise to yourself to always choose joy . . . despite whatever is going on. People often accuse others of "making" them feel a certain way. But guess what— that's a myth! No one can control how you feel. You always get to choose your emotions and how you respond to stuff. So if someone spreads a rumor about you, do you knee-jerk react in anger or offer kindness? When your friend 'fesses up to a mistake, will you judge her or be the gal who uplifts her?

The other fab part about joy? It spreads out faster and wider than any rumor or dark influence. Let it start with you. Flash a big smile at that store clerk—even if she's rude!

Let the sea resound, and all that is in it; let the fields be jubilant, and everything in them! Let the trees of the forest sing, let them sing for joy before the Lord.

1 Chronicles 16:32–33 NIV

Reflect

Jesus tells us to keep His commandments and abide in His love so that we might find joy! The next time you feel a little blue, gently turn your mood by focusing on anything that brings a smile—a pet hamster, your funky new socks, the heart emoji your friend texted today.

Respond

Journal at least five fun ways you might find joy. Then actually do a few—or all!—of them this week. Start your checklist right here:

_____

_____

_____

I'm so happy that even when things go wrong, I can find joy in you. Thank you for never leaving my side and reminding me that you are all I need in this crazy world!

Mean girls are spreading rumors about me.

Have you ever had someone spread a bad rumor about you that was a complete lie? It's not a great feeling to know that someone is being negative and talking about you behind your back. In the end, we can't control what other people do. But this doesn't take away the pain we might feel!

Everyone has been affected by gossip at one point or another. Even the biggest celebrities in the world have had something negative said about them and have probably had their feelings hurt. But just like the hottest fashion and TikTok trends go away after a while, so do rumors! It's out with the old and in with the new when the "next best thing" hits the scene. Although this doesn't take away the fact that hearing rumors about yourself hurts, you still have the choice to decide if you will let it affect you or not. You can choose to stand firm in the confident, smart, and bold girl that you are, and ignore the haters around you.

No one is protected from other people's opinions—even your own. While it's okay to have opinions, we should be mindful of gossiping with friends. Do you find yourself talking down about others with your girlfriends, or are you choosing to be positive? Being conscious of how you speak about others when they are not present not only shows others your light, but also can inspire other girls to be better!

Our words have power (see Proverbs 18:21 and Mark 11:23). God gives us the power and authority to use our faith to do great things. If your words have power, why would you use that power to hurt someone?

The words that come out of our mouths are ultimately reflections of what is in our hearts. If pain lives in your heart, pain is what will flow from your lips. If joy lives in your heart, positivity and encouragement will flow from your lips. Jesus wants us to spread His love throughout the Earth—how can we do that if we use the power of our words to gossip?

Do not use harmful words, but only helpful words, the kind that build up and provide what is needed, so that what you say will do good to those who hear you.

Ephesians 4:29 GNT

Reflect

Take the chitchat challenge: From now on, try your best to say *only* kind words about people—even celebrities, even people you don't like. If you're tempted to say something negative or unkind, instead . . . zip it.

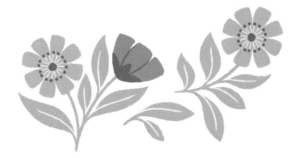

Respond

Think of someone who has been the target of unfair gossip, and say a prayer for that person. Pray also for those who spread the rumors. Write your prayers down here:

_____

_____

_____

_____

_____

_____

_____

_____

_____

It's true, God. I've been hurt before by someone's mean words and it doesn't feel good at all. I don't ever want to hurt someone that way, so can you help me always be the bigger person?

I want to be a better listener.

We have two ears and one mouth. Maybe that's so we can listen more than we speak! Your caregiver may say, "You never listen." And you might feel that *they* never listen to *you*—maybe you're convinced they don't process a word you say. But do *you* pay attention to your own listening skills?

Perhaps you have been in a situation in which you spoke too soon . . . or talked too much. Maybe a friend told you something, and you responded in a way that came off as insensitive. And then the more you tried to smooth it out, the more tangled your words got. And then you realized you had misunderstood what your friend was trying to tell you all along. Take a moment and shush it! Learn to be a good listener.

You do a lot of listening in your life, in school, while watching TV, when streaming music. Just as you can be choosy about your words, actions, and behavior, you also get to decide how you feel about what you hear. Are you going to get worked up over what someone posted on social media, or will you listen instead to your own intuition about what God says?

You've often heard the phrase "think before you speak," right? That's good advice, and similarly it's not a bad idea to "listen before you respond." It forces you to slow down and process what you are hearing . . . to truly listen.

When Jesus traveled to different cities with His disciples to preach, large crowds came to hear Him. Even though He spent a lot of time speaking, He spent just as much time in solitude and prayer, listening to God. He wants the same thing for you!

Anyone who has an ear should listen to what the Spirit says to the churches. I will give the victor the right to eat from the tree of life, which is in God's paradise.

Revelation 2:7 HCSB

Reflect

When you talk to God, He listens. He hears you—that's a promise! So have a conversation with Him. Share your thoughts, and His response will come in perfect timing. Now, it's time for *you* to listen. Notice His little "nods"; hear His "nudges."

Respond

Sit in a circle with family or friends for a gab session about how you can be better listeners. Use the lines below, or a blank sheet of paper, to play a classic listening game. Write down a favorite short verse from the Bible—don't tell it! Whisper it into the ear of the person next to you. That person whispers to the next person, and so on. The last person says the verse out loud. Does the verse match up to what's written on the paper? Probably not!

_____

_____

_____

_____

_____

_____

_____

_____

_____

_____

_____

_____

_____

_____

_____

God, thank you for listening to all of my prayers. Thank you for being a friend to rely on. I find so much peace and joy in knowing you listen when I call! Amen.

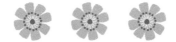

Social media is stressing me out.

Can you imagine having to wait weeks or months to hear the latest news from your bestie? In the time we live in, thanks to technology and social media, it's so much easier to keep up with all the important people in our lives than it was in the past. And at its best, social media is a fun way to stay connected with friends and family and discover new points of view.

But while social media is lots of fun, it's not always as it seems! What you see on your feed—the girl with the perfect selfie angle and flawless skin—is more times than not heavily edited to look almost perfect. I mean, that's the goal, right? To look like you have the best of the best and the perfect life? Wrong! It's all a deceptive illusion that can sometimes make you feel like you aren't enough.

People tend to only post what makes them "look" the best and don't like to share the reality of it all. Even though you always see your favorite celebrity post about the awesome life they have doesn't mean that they don't have bad days, too. Just because that IG model seems like she always has perfect skin doesn't mean that she doesn't gets zits sometimes, too! We often forget that on the other side of the screen there are humans just like us.

If you find yourself starting to feel insecure because of the things you see on your feed, it might be time to think about how much time you're actually spending online. It's so easy to get sucked into the vacuum and start binge-watching your feed, and before you know it, hours have passed! Consider setting a time limit for yourself when it comes to enjoying social media so that you don't forget about the important things, like connection with friends and family face-to-face.

Though we all go through the cycle of comparing ourselves to others, it's important to understand that social media does not define who we are—God does. Even if it feels like the world is judging what you look like, God says that you are strong and courageous.

The next time you log onto your social media account, make a commitment to not compare yourself to what you see on your feed. At the end of the day, God reminds us that we are not alone in this journey of life.

> *"Everything is permissible for me," but not everything is helpful. "Everything is permissible for me," but I will not be brought under the control of anything.*
>
> **1 Corinthians 6:12 HCSB**

Reflect

How can you spread love on your social media pages? Perhaps "share" or "like" a friend's posted achievement—she won that poetry contest, yay! Post inspirational quotes about strong women in the Bible. Talk to a teacher or caregiver about using social media to kick off a positive campaign, such as collecting school supplies for kids who need them.

Respond

Use the space below to draft a list of things you love to do that don't involve social media. Unplug for a day to ride your bike, plant some sunflower seeds, or play a board game with the sibs. What else do you want to do?

_____

_____

_____

_____

_____

_____

Sometimes I feel like I am broken, but you say that I am whole. Sometimes I feel alone but, God, then I remember you are near me always. You give me hope when I feel hopeless. Thank you. Amen.

Shhhh, don't tell anyone my secret!

Have you ever shared something personal with a close friend? Maybe you and your siblings share secrets with one another, and you trust that they won't tell anyone. But there might be secrets you have not shared with *anyone*—things only you know and hold close because it feels safer that way or because you don't want anyone to judge you. Perhaps you have a slew of secret fears, wishes, likes, and dislikes. Or maybe you have a secret that feels shameful.

But you really have no secrets, because God sees and knows everything. He is omniscient, which means He is all-knowing. God knows the deepest darkest secrets of our hearts even if we have not voiced them to anyone. Does the thought of that send a chill through your spine? Does it feel like you have the eye of a super-spy on you? Well, don't fret, because guess what—God sees it all . . . and *loves* you. He knows the way you think, and He understands every part of you— even when you don't understand.

He also knows your emotions. You are keeping pesky secrets when you choose not to honestly express how you feel. Whatever you are feeling, you can always rest in the arms of the Comforter. He is always listening, and He knows how to free you if you have a secret that feels painful. Do you want to hide . . . or seek?

Sure, it can feel odd to place your trust in this great mystery known as God—something that sometimes feels so secretive in itself. But the Bible promises, "keep on asking and it will be given to you." So ask away, and discover what divine secrets will be revealed to *you!*

> *There are some things the Lord our God has kept secret. But there are some things he has let us know. These things belong to us and our children forever.*

Deuteronomy 29:29 ICB

Reflect

How can you invite God into the secret places in your heart? It's usually easier to connect with God in stillness, so start a new daily routine. Take ten minutes each morning to meditate. If you don't have time in the morning, do it later in the day. But no excuses—nobody doesn't have ten minutes to spare! Just sit quietly, and still your mind. Search your Bible for scripture verses about meditation.

Respond

Write down some of your secrets in the space provided, and spend some quiet time in prayer to share them with God. If you're worried about your little brother reading this like a diary, come up with a secret written code that only you know how to crack.

_____

_____

_____

_____

_____

_____

_____

_____

_____

_____

> God, even though I have deep secrets that I don't want to share with anyone, I know that you love me no matter what. You know me and you love me—even when I forget to love myself. Thank you for your perfect love. Amen.

What does respect mean?

———

Respect is about how you regard someone and ultimately how you treat that person—and that includes yourself! How many times have you heard "treat others the way you want to be treated"? Well, this saying actually comes from the Bible. That's what is meant when it reads, "love thy neighbor as thyself." Jesus wants us to respect *everyone*—no exceptions.

Respecting others means being compassionate, polite, and kind, which are all ways Jesus lived His life. He sat and ate with beggars or people who were poor and didn't have money to care for themselves or family. But He also sat with some of the most influential people, such as priests and kings. Regardless of others' social status, Jesus treated everyone with the same respect. You can do the same!

It is also important to respect yourself—and to expect others to show you respect. You are God's daughter, and it's important to know your true worth. Don't say things to belittle yourself. Even casually with friends, if you say, "Oh, I'm stupid!" or "Sheesh, I hate my nose," you're not respecting who God made you to be. And if someone treats you with anything less than basic respect, don't slump over in gloom or defeat. Hold your head high, stand firm, and simply say, "Respect, please."

When you respect yourself and others, you are living like Jesus lived and, ultimately, that is what He wants. Start right now. Look in the mirror, make eye contact with yourself, and say, "I love and respect you—I really do." And mean it!

*Live as servants of God. Show respect for all
people. Love the brothers and sisters of God's
family. Respect God. Honor the king.*

1 Peter 2:16–17 ICB

Reflect

In your quiet time, maybe before your daily meditation, ask God
to help you understand how you can respect yourself more.
How can you show others more respect—your caregivers, other
family members, teachers, or friends? God will guide you, so
follow His lead.

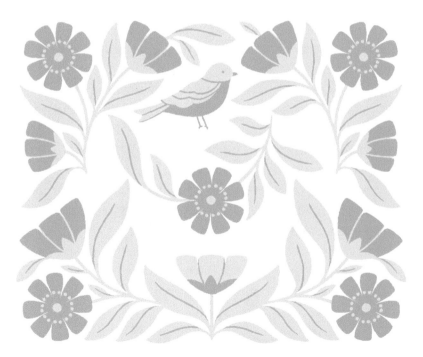

Respond

You've heard that popular song about respect, right? Gospel and soul singer Aretha Franklin made the song a hit, spelling it as she belted it out: "R-E-S-P-E-C-T." In the lines below, write an acrostic poem. You'll see the word "RESPECT" in capital letters vertically down the left margin. The first sentence or line of your poem begins with "R," the second line "E," the next "S," then "P," and so on.

R _____

E _____

S _____

P _____

E _____

C _____

T

> I ultimately want to make you proud, God, but sometimes people upset me and it's hard to even think about respect for myself and others. Can you guide me in the right direction?

How can I spend time with God?

Worship is one of the most beautiful things about faith. Worship is more than just singing a song or praying—worship is a way of life as a believer. Everything you do has the potential to be an act of worship toward God. We worship because God loves it and because it's how we express our love to the Father.

The cool thing is that worship can be so many different things. I learned how to worship God in my sport by honoring Him in my performance. I no longer competed to beat the person next to me. I performed and gave my best to show God that I am thankful for the gift of athletic ability. Or maybe you like to express yourself in art or music. You can worship God in your art or your skills by honoring who He is and how He made you!

Although worship can be enjoyed publicly with friends or your church community, it can also be fulfilling when done in private. Spending time alone with God opens the door for powerful and intimate worship with your Creator. I've experienced some of the most peaceful moments when I chose to worship alone in my room uninterrupted, and I've had similar experiences at church gatherings.

There's no right or wrong way to worship. It feels so good to share your faith and beliefs with friends who care! But try to be mindful of those around you who might not share the same beliefs, or who might not be ready to hear about God. You should always be true to yourself and your faith, but you can choose the form of worship that makes the most sense in the moment. Maybe before lunch at school you might bow your head in blessing, or you might thank God silently for the A you just scored on that test. Or you might pray together with a teammate who you know shares your faith before the big game.

How can worship look so different in different situations? Because worship is the act of honoring God. If we honor God in our sports, our words, our songs, or our poems, we're worshipping God!

Let us worship and bow down; let us kneel before the Lord our Maker. For He is our God, and we are the people of His pasture, and the sheep of His hand.

Psalm 95:6–7 NKJV

Reflect

What ways do you worship God? Do you talk openly about your faith, or do you prefer to have a more personal relationship with Him? Or maybe you're somewhere in between!

Respond

Make a list below of some of your favorite worship songs, and sing them out loud—even if it's just in the shower!

_____

_____

_____

_____

_____

_____

_____

_____

_____

_____

_____

_____

_____

It's so cool to know that I can sing a song, write a
poem, or even draw a picture and you embrace
it as worship! Thank you for loving me just as
I am, God!

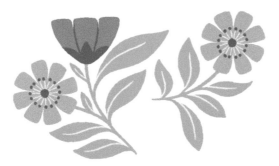

How can I serve God and others?

We know that Jesus's entire life was dedication to serving others. Jesus wants us to live our lives for His glory—He wants us to love and serve others! But where does that fit in between home, school, sports or band practice, and trying to keep up the rest of your life in the meantime?

Service is not limited to volunteering at your church or school. Service can look like doing your chores and keeping your room tidy out of respect and adoration for your caregivers. Service can look like using your gifts and talents to lift up other people. Do you like to write? Use that gift to write words that encourage other people. Do you like to make art? Create something that invokes inspiration and creativity for others!

While serving others is a major part of faith, so is service to self. Service to self doesn't mean giving yourself what you want when you want it—it means taking care of yourself, because God wants you to be well. God sees you as precious, so you should care for yourself in that way.

Let's say you're working on a group project and your partner needs help, but you have to finish your work, too. If you're grumpy because you skipped your snack at recess, you might be less happy about helping your partner. When you take the time to address your own needs, you put yourself in a position to give to others from a place of wholeness instead of from a place that's unbalanced.

At the end of the day, Jesus wants us to be a reflection of Him, and we cannot do that without loving, serving, and giving to others.

Offer hospitality to one another without grumbling. Each of you should use whatever gift you have received to serve others, as faithful stewards of God's grace.

1 Peter 4:9–10 NIV

Reflect

Think back on a time when you helped someone and how it made you feel. Then think about a time that somebody helped you. The feelings are sort of the same, aren't they? Helping others is a win-win.

Respond

Ask a caregiver or teacher for a way you can volunteer in your neighborhood or at school. Maybe your church needs a helper in the nursery or kitchen. Some schools require students to take part in volunteer work. Even if yours doesn't, you can still offer to volunteer. Check your local library, too—they might need a hand, and if not, a librarian can help you find opportunities for service in your community. Use the space below to keep notes.

_____

_____

_____

_____

_____

_____

_____

_____

_____

_____

_____

_____

I have to admit—sometimes I enjoy helping
and giving back to others but other times not
so much. Why does it get hard sometimes?
Please show me new ways to serve those around
me! Amen.

Grown-ups think they know it all. Do they really?

You probably have embarrassing memories from the past, things you'd do differently if you'd known what you know now. We all do! In order to become wiser, we sometimes have to experience pain from hard lessons. Having wisdom is a beautiful thing, but the first time we run into a problem it's hard to know how to handle it.

Have you ever had a special person you look up to, like a coach or a teacher? Think about why you look up to them. Maybe you aspire to be like them when you grow up, or maybe they always know what to say to help you muddle through confusion. This is what it is like to experience wisdom.

God has put people in our lives—like our parents—to help guide us. In your lifetime you will meet teachers, coaches, and sometimes even complete strangers who will share wisdom that helps you grow. Hold on to these ideas in your heart. There will be one day you'll remember what God or someone else spoke to you, and that wisdom will help you deal with a tough situation.

While adults have had lots of experiences and can often give you advice, they don't always have all the answers. For example, you might come across an adult who is disrespectful toward a group of people, maybe because of what they look like or who they are. While it is important to always respect elders, it is also important to tell what is *from* God and what is not. God loves all his children, so anything hateful is probably not of God.

Think about your wisdom as a tool. As you grow with God, your wisdom becomes a sharper tool that will help you!

If any of you lack wisdom, you should pray to God, who will give it to you; because God gives graciously and generously to all. But when you pray, you must believe and not doubt at all.

James 1:5–6 GNT

Reflect

Is there a celebrity, such as an activist or politician, you look up to and want to learn from? The most famous person in history to live wholly in faith was Jesus! God sent Jesus to be a shining example. So if you want to keep your eyes on the wise, look to His teachings.

Respond

Look up the word "mentor" in the dictionary, and write its definition here. Then make a list of ideal qualities and characteristics you'd like to see in a mentor. Read the list back to yourself. Does it bring to mind anyone you already know? If not, trust that God will bring the perfect mentor to you at just the right time.

_____

_____

_____

_____

_____

_____

_____

_____

_____

_____

_____

_____

_____

_____

God, thank you for allowing me to have wisdom simply by asking you. Will you help me humble my heart and listen and accept knowledge of your wise ways? I know you will. Amen.

What's the best way to spend my allowance?

———

This world, for better or worse, operates on money. It's needed to live, eat, and buy cool stuff. Practically speaking, you need money to meet the basic needs of life—and that's not a bad thing! It is always important to consider, though, how you look at and manage money.

Many scriptures say not to be consumed with materialistic things such as money (see 1 Timothy 6:10, Hebrews 13:5, Proverbs 13:11, and Matthew 6:24). When Jesus walked the earth, He reminded everyone that they should love people more than they love money. He taught people not to be consumed with the ways of this world.

At the same time, it's important to have faith in the abundance God brings. And it's also key to be generous with what you have. Think about how you spend your allowance or birthday money. Do you first run to the store to drop all your cash on new stuff? Or do you first set aside a portion to share, to donate, or to spend on gifts for others? There is no wrong answer here, and you shouldn't feel any guilt for wanting to buy candy or toys or whatever your heart desires. But giving generously can warm your heart more than a solo shopping spree.

No matter what, try not to fall into the trap of buying things just to feel cool or fit in. Nothing can make you feel more a part of something than the love of God.

Give to others, and God will give to you. Indeed, you will receive a full measure, a generous helping, poured into your hands—all that you can hold. The measure you use for others is the one that God will use for you.

Luke 6:38 GNT

Reflect

Shopping can be loads of fun! But do you sometimes buy things to fill a void in your heart? No amount of money—or stuff!—can give you the riches that God provides. He flows pure love to you and through you, and your only job is to line up with it. "Thank you" will do.

Respond

Money is often associated with abundance. But God gives abundantly in many ways—through friendships, nature, pets, sunrises, and so much more. Make a list in the space provided of all the ways you feel richly blessed.

_____

_____

_____

_____

_____

_____

_____

_____

_____

_____

_____

_____

_____

_____

_____

_____

_____

_____

> Jesus, sometimes I like to buy things because it makes me feel cool. I know that no matter what I buy, you say that I am already whole, loved, and pure in your name. Thank you for your grace and kindness! Amen.

So many things to do, so little time.

Sometimes it can be hard keeping up with everything on your schedule. You've got school, friends, band practice, chess club, orthodontist appointments. Even weekends, when you want to just hang out, can get hectic—maybe you go to church with your parents or you go to see family. Life often serves up competing priorities, and sometimes your weekly agenda is out of your control. For example, it's unlikely your caregivers are going to let you skip school to, say, skip rope—your activity of choice.

For activities in which you do have free rein, it's really helpful to make priorities. About each of the things you need to cross off your list, you might be thinking, *Why does this matter?* Well, when you prioritize, you decide what goes at the top of your to-do list. You decide what matters the most, so your priorities reflect what you most care about. But Jesus doesn't want us to be swamped with competing priorities. He wants to be top priority in your life. It's *not* that He has a big attention-craving ego. It's because He knows if you turn to Him first, He can help guide your day so everything falls into place in a perfect unfolding of events.

The Bible says to seek first the kingdom of God (see the scripture passage on page 39) and also that each moment is "a new creation," a clean slate, so to speak! So before worrying about what's for breakfast or what clothes to wear, line up with God. Make a promise to love others, be compassionate, and honor all of God's creations. Then pay attention to how your day plays out.

> *The thing you should want most is God's kingdom and doing what God wants. Then all these other things you need will be given to you.*

Matthew 6:33 ICB

Reflect

When you remember to put God first, everything else falls into place perfectly. How can you better prioritize your relationship with God? Make yourself a promise to connect with Him every morning. Greet Him first thing when the sun peers through your bedroom windows. Say, "Hello, God!"

Respond

Gather your family and agree on a priority list of chores in your household. Use the space below to outline weekly tasks. At the tippy-top of that list, include time for getting to know Jesus. Do you know what Jesus told His friends Martha and Mary—they were sisters—about washing dishes? Break out your Bible and turn to Luke 10:38–42.

_____

_____

_____

_____

_____

_____

_____

_____

_____

_____

_____

_____

God, sometimes I get off track and forget my priorities, but thank you for your kindness, wisdom, and grace! Help me to be wise with where I am focusing my time and energy. Amen.

I worry so much!

Simply put, anxiety is a constant mental state of worrying. To better imagine what anxiety is like, think about a large ball made of hundreds of rubber bands. When someone deals with anxiety, their thoughts are like those rubber bands—deeply mixed up with one another and pulled in many directions.

Little kids are often breezy and carefree, but as we age, we all start to worry more. But how do some of us get to a point of constant worry? Well, some stress over things like grades. And others struggle with issues like parents who bicker or a pet that's sick. Everyone's situation is different, but it's not unusual for people to, well, time travel: They brood over the past and also try to predict the future. When you worry about what's to come or something that has already happened, you remove yourself from the power of the present moment.

Jesus very clearly tells us, "do not worry," promising that God will "meet all your needs" (see Matthew 6:34 and Philippians 4:19). When you allow anxiety to take over, it steers you away from the beauty of being conscious *right now*. Why worry when you know God will provide the perfect solution to every perceived problem?

As someone who lives with anxiety, I can tell you that through prayer it is very possible to overcome the negative thoughts you have for yourself. If you find yourself in a fray or funk, you *will* make it through. With the support of the Holy Spirit, you can summon the strength that lies deep within your soul to take charge of your thoughts and emotions. (If you are overwhelmed by anxiety, you may also want to seek care from a licensed mental health practitioner, perhaps one who shares your faith.) Don't be discouraged, because when you trust in the Lord, He will direct your path.

Here are three simple steps to help you when you take off on the worry train:

1. First take a moment for a deep breath, and just count to ten. This forces you to stop head-tripping and brings you back to the present.

2. Next, write down anything that is worrying you. Are you concerned about a test coming up? Anxious about the health of a family member? Write your thoughts down to clarify what is in your mind.

3. Finally, take your concerns to God. Tell Him exactly what you are worried about, and let Him know that you trust His solution. Ask Him to still your heart and mind and to give you wisdom and peace about the situation.

No worrisome thought will withstand that triple-threat approach! There's strength in acknowledging that God is your Redeemer.

Humble yourselves, therefore, under the mighty hand of God, so that He may exalt you at the proper time, casting all your care on Him, because He cares about you.

1 Peter 5:6–7 HCSB

Reflect

Why worry when you can choose faith instead? Um . . .
enough said!

Respond

Write down a list of your main concerns below. At the end of
your list write, "God, I'm giving all of the above to you!" Then
spend time alone to pray with God, asking Him to settle your
heart and guide you. Now what? Just trust.

_____

_____

_____

_____

_____

_____

Thank you for being a loving and gracious Father.
Because you care for me, I know that all of life's
worries don't even compare to how you have my
back. Thank you! Amen.

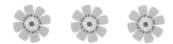

How can I believe without seeing?

We all have little things that we believe in faith for every day. To have faith in something is to trust and be confident in it. You might have faith that the sun will rise tomorrow morning, or you might have faith that your family loves you. But faith in God is different, and bigger, than all other kinds of faith!

Our faith in God means we trust in Him even if we can't see firsthand evidence of God's grace. The whole idea of faith is that we believe in our hearts. We know within ourselves that God is here with us.

There was a woman in the Bible who had a health problem that no one could heal (see Luke 8:43–48). She went to many different doctors and spent all the money that she had in the hope that someone could heal her.

One day she heard that Jesus would be coming to her town. She was so desperate to meet him that when Jesus and his disciples were walking through the town, she forced her way through the thick crowd and she touched the edge of his clothing. She believed that if she could simply touch Jesus that she would be healed. That is strong faith!

Jesus immediately stopped and asked, "Who touched me?" He felt that someone with astounding faith had touched Him. Trembling, the woman confessed that it was she who had touched Him. Jesus spoke that her faith had healed her!

Why does all of this matter? Because of the woman's belief in things not seen. The woman didn't know anything except that

Jesus would be nearby. Her faith gave her the strength to push through the crowd and her faith in Jesus ultimately yielded her being healed.

One of the ways that our faith can be energized is by remembering times that God has been faithful. Can you think about a time when you saw something miraculous happen? Maybe your dog got really sick but ended up recovering when you didn't think they were going to make it. How did you feel? What were your thoughts? I can only imagine that at first you were scared about whatever the situation was, but as things shifted you were probably amazed. Sometimes choosing to believe and have faith might seem crazy, but it is the root of our relationship with Jesus. Why? Because although you cannot physically see God, you still believe that He is real and that He loves you. It's in this concept of believing in things not seen where we find the most challenging yet fulfilling experiences that draw us closer to God.

Without faith it is impossible to please God, because anyone who comes to Him must believe that He exists and that He rewards those who earnestly seek Him.

Hebrews 11:6 NIV

Reflect

How can you practice having more faith in an area that you struggle with? Gather your family for a group discussion. Ask everyone to share about a time when God has shown Himself faithful.

Respond

Open your Bible and read Hebrews 11. Faith is about believing in what you cannot see with your eyes. It's about using your imagination! Think of something in your life that could be better. But be thankful for the current situation, since it inspires you to imagine an improvement. Write an essay below that details not how things are, but how you want them to be. And then stay in faith of God's perfect plan for you.

_____

_____

_____

_____

_____

_____

Gosh—faith can be a little confusing to me. Is it really true that I just have to believe and then I am saved? Is it really that simple? Help me understand, God!

I want to be a leader!

Sometimes it might feel like if you're not pushing the limit, you aren't going to be successful in life. It might seem like you're falling short if you don't have all wins on the field or lots of classmates who want to be your friend. This might be how you feel in the moment, but it isn't true.

Instead of believing what the world says about us, what if we chose to trust that Jesus believes in us? What if we went out into the world and spread more of His love? Ultimately, that is why we were all created! We were created to know Jesus and to make Him known on this side of heaven. But how can we lead a life like Christ did if we don't believe that He trusts in us?

In order to lead a life like the Lord did, we must first decide that we believe His word. God's word says that we should love our neighbors as we love ourselves. That means: When a bully or a friend says something mean to you or someone else, don't respond in anger. But be sure you stand up for what's right with grace and love. Hold your own sense of self-respect and respect your own values, but without creating a grudge. You should forgive!

Let no one despise your youth, but be an example to the believers in word, in conduct, in love, in spirit, in faith, in purity.

1 Timothy 4:12 NKJV

Reflect

Some people are natural-born leaders—others, not so much. If you have a tendency to be more of a follower, that's okay, too. But be aware of what and whom you are following. Do you really want to copycat the "too cool for rules" crowd? Or would you rather stick with true-blue friends who show integrity? It's your call!

Respond

Whether your tendency is to lead or follow, challenge yourself to take the reins on something that's important to you. Maybe you could run for president of a club or take charge of a big project in youth group. Use the space provided to make an outline of some initial ideas.

_____

_____

_____

_____

_____

God, sometimes it is hard to live a life as a leader for Christ. Sometimes I don't want to lead—I want to follow. I know that your truth is what's best for me, so I will follow you and rely on your Spirit to guide me. Amen.

Fear can't stop me.

Feeling afraid is the worst! Everyone has fears. Some people are afraid of heights and don't like going to adventure parks. Some people are afraid of snakes or mice—yuck! But sometimes fear isn't as straightforward as disliking animals or roller coasters. Maybe you're afraid of trying out for the cheerleading or soccer team. Maybe you're afraid of having a conversation with a teacher about an unfair grade. You might even be afraid to invite your crush to a party. The fear you feel might be so strong that it cripples you from making a decision or taking action.

Not letting fear stop you can be difficult, but there are ways to overcome it. First things first: You can't process something you don't acknowledge. This means that you have to understand and accept the emotion you feel! Sit with it, feel it, and try to understand why you feel the way that you do. Once you acknowledge it, you can make a plan. Decide in your heart and mind that you will move forward and take action. When you do, celebrate yourself! Once you have that conversation with your teacher, or show up to the soccer tryout, give yourself a pat on the back for being bold and taking a leap of faith. Once you start taking small steps, you'll feel better looking fear in the eye and standing tall.

Fear is one of those things that will always be lurking in the background of every decision. Sometimes, if we fall into the fear-based mindset, we'll keep ourselves in our comfort zones. It's absolutely okay to be afraid! And to be completely honest, it's in those moments of fear where we have a beautiful opportunity to draw near to God.

No matter what, people will let us down because, well, they are people. Human beings are not perfect and in one way or another we can and will fall short. Have your caregivers or friends ever let you down before? I'm sure they have! But that doesn't mean that they don't love and care for you. It just means that they are human and have fallen short.

The beauty that's found in fear is that no matter what, God doesn't leave our side. He delights in being in communion with us! He smiles when we lean on Him instead of letting fear cripple us. His love is perfect and never-ending. God is a good God and nothing can ever change that!

Remember that I commanded you to be strong and brave. So don't be afraid. The Lord your God will be with you everywhere you go.

Joshua 1:9 ICB

Reflect

Fear is not your friend! Fear can serve as a helpful signal that something is "off," so don't ignore it. But at the same time, don't stay stuck in a fearful mindset. That will trip you up every time. This is why it's often recommended that you "face your fears." Once you confront whatever terrifies you, the fear tends to disappear. Poof!

Respond

Spend some time pondering your fears, and think of some ways you can choose faith instead. If you're afraid of the water, perhaps you'll consider swimming lessons. Because your knees buckle at the thought of talking in front of a group, debate club might do you good. You're scared to tell your caregivers how you feel about something? Use the space provided to write them a letter. If you're feeling really brave, share it with them.

_____

_____

_____

_____

_____

_____

God, sometimes I do get scared. People have let me down in my life before, so at times I assume the worst in certain situations. Can you help me begin choosing faith over fear? You're the best! Amen.

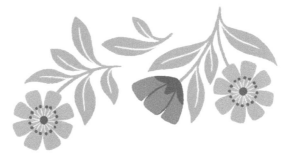

How can I remember to stay grateful?

Gratitude has everything to do with thankfulness, appreciation, and being glad! I'm sure you can think of a time when you felt really excited and thankful for something that happened in your life. Maybe you got exactly what you wanted for Christmas or your birthday or maybe a friend did something special for you. I can only imagine that your heart was overflowing with joy and gratitude, which left you feeling more alive than ever!

But life isn't always exciting and perfect, right? There might be a time when you just can't seem to do well in one of your classes. It seems like no matter how much you study you just can't seem to understand the information to get a passing grade! Maybe you're upset because you think your allowance is too low or maybe you play sports and this season your team just isn't performing at its best. Practices are hard and you guys just can't seem to win any game or competition—how frustrating!

Although you will go through difficult times, it's up to you to shift your attitude and perspective. How? Instead of choosing to be upset about what you lack or don't have, you can choose to be grateful about what you do have. Choosing an attitude of gratitude and appreciation not only puts you in a better mental state but also opens the door for more positivity to come into your life.

The key to embracing gratitude is understanding that it is not only a feeling but also a choice. Think about it. If you have a sour attitude because you think your allowance is too low, that feeling is not going to instantly change. You have to make the *choice* to change your attitude and perspective, and then your emotions will catch up—meaning that even if you don't feel grateful in the moment, eventually you will if you continue to choose to be appreciative.

When you choose to have an attitude of gratitude, you are forcing yourself to focus on things that you have instead of what you *think* you lack. Your circumstances can shift when you stop focusing on negativity and instead set your eyes and heart on seeing the beauty of what you have. When you do, it strengthens your faith. You are never alone, because God is with you. Even though tough times will come, you will make it to the other side with the help of God and your positive attitude.

But life is hard, right? You're probably thinking that there is no way someone can be positive and grateful in every situation possible. This is where your faith comes in! Just like you are going to experience amazing and joyful moments in your life, you will equally experience hard and painful moments. Maybe your dog died or a loved one is very ill and passed away. Those are very real and very painful emotions that are completely valid and are something that you should process. But you shouldn't stay in that mental space forever. There comes a moment when you have to make the conscious decision to choose joy and hope over every other painful emotion you might feel.

The key to gratitude is staying rooted in Christ and what the word of God says. When we are rooted, we are grounded and planted in a solid foundation of truth. Think about a house. When it's being built, its foundation is made of concrete so when a strong storm comes it won't collapse. That's the same thing that happens when you are rooted in the word of God. When hard seasons pass through your life, you won't fall down, because your foundation is on the solid rock and truth of Jesus Christ.

> *Be joyful always, pray at all times, be thankful in all circumstances. This is what God wants from you in your life in union with Christ Jesus.*
>
> **1 Thessalonians 5:16–18 GNT**

Reflect

Maybe you've heard it a million times, but it is worth repeating. Gratitude is an attitude! Feeling a lack of appreciation? That's an easy fix! Shift your thinking to focus on things you love, no matter how big or small.

Respond

When you're out and about this week, notice the things you appreciate. As you walk outside in nature and even around your home, give thanks to God for how He provides. What are you thankful for in your life? Write about it.

_____

_____

_____

_____

_____

_____

_____

_____

_____

_____

_____

_____

_____

_____

_____

Sometimes things really upset me and it's hard to stay grateful about the things I already have in my life. I want to do better, and with your help I know that I can!

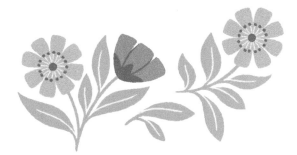

God, why is there so much hate in the world?

———

Unfortunately, violence and hate take place all over the world. Violence isn't always necessarily physical—some mental or emotional wrongdoings toward others might be considered violent, like maliciously hacking a website. Violent threats might be made against a person or community online. Regardless of the way it's expressed, violence results in pain. But many rise up in the wake of violence—for instance, when neighbors form a unifying bond as they come together to heal from a local tragedy such as a shooting.

These might be some scary thoughts, but it's important not to deny your feelings when experiencing the pinch of negativity. Emotions that are held in or ignored do not go away. They fester and smolder, and they seep out sideways in your daily life. For example, if that boy on the football team talked to you with a foul mouth, you might say, "Oh, that didn't bother me one little bit." And maybe it didn't, which is great!

But if the boy's verbal attacks actually did get under your skin, and you have not processed those emotions, there's a chance you will be reluctant to trust other boys and judge collectively. Don't do that! *Feel* your not-so-fuzzy feelings. You can process them privately or tell a trusted friend or adult—but then give them to God. Don't stay stuck in emotional muck.

What, then, should you do when violence or abuse is brought to light? The best place to start is to look at Jesus and how He lived His life. He constantly chose peace and love over "repaying" the many people who treated Him poorly. Jesus suffered the ultimate sacrifice because He loves us. He endured the most violent physical torture as He trekked to the cross. He was beaten, whipped, and spit on. And what did He say? "Father, forgive them for they do not know what they do." How incredibly mind-blowing is that? In the face of adversity, violence, and immense pain and suffering, your loving Savior asked for forgiveness for His abusers. That is true love.

And what of you? Do you ever lean toward violence? Do you sometimes feel like swearing at your sister for stealing your sweaters, or bopping your brother on the head when he belches in front of your friends to the tune of the national anthem? Regardless of what is going on in your world, violence is never the answer. Even if you have experienced a great injustice and feel as though reacting aggressively is valid, you get to choose: violence and pain or love and forgiveness?

Don't argue with others for no reason when they have never done you any harm. Don't be jealous of violent people or decide to act as they do.

Proverbs 3:30–31 GNT

Reflect

There are boatloads of benefits to choosing love over anger! Think about a time when you didn't act in a loving way but instead gave in to anger. What was the outcome? How could you have chosen love instead?

Respond

Journal about something that gets you particularly peeved. Pour out your feelings in the space provided. Scribble if it helps! That's right—show your anger. Yes, ultimately choose love. But first express your feelings, in such a way that you own your feelings without emotionally dumping on others. Then shake it off.

_____

_____

_____

_____

_____

Jesus, I've got a bunch of questions about the violence I've seen happen. I know you will help me understand how to process these emotions.

I want to be the best on the team!

Growing up as an avid athlete, sports were everything to me. I ran track, did gymnastics, and cheered competitively. Like most athletes, I was obsessed with perfecting my craft. Endless practice and game hours were spent doing what I loved most. But it got to a point where my sports performance was how I measured my worth. If I didn't perform well or my team didn't win, I felt angry and worthless, like I had let my team down.

God blesses you with this awesome activity called sports because He loves you. He likes to see you use your athletic ability, and He loves that it brings you and many others joy— participants *and* spectators. But your worth is not found in how well you perform in your sport. God already names you as worthy of His love.

So how can you use your sport as an opportunity to commune with God? Instead of playing for the approval of friends or family or fans, play for an audience of one: Jesus! He is not concerned with whether you make the winning basket, or score the most points, or beat your best running time. He just wants you to have fun with it! What matters is that you have the opportunity to glorify God through wins and even losses. Are you a sour person if your team tanks, or are you the one to say, "Hey, we win some and lose some. Thank you, God, for the chance to play!"

Anyone who competes as an athlete does not receive the victor's crown except by competing according to the rules.

2 Timothy 2:5 NIV

Reflect

How can you use your sport to worship God? At church or Christian schools, students often pray to kick off athletic competitions and other activities. If you're in public school, however, it might not be ordinary to pray before a game. But, hey, you can break those rules and say a prayer—sort of. No one can tell you you can't worship the Lord, so recite your prayers silently or with a teammate. Game on!

Respond

Make a list of ways you can lift others up on your sports team as a leader in Christ. For example, invite teammates to join you in silent prayer before and after a game—even if it's during phys ed class—or come up with a team cheer that gives faith-based values a big shout-out!

_____

_____

_____

_____

_____

_____

_____

_____

_____

_____

_____

_____

_____

_____

_____

God, thank you for the gift of sports and for giving me athletic ability. Continue to show me how I can worship you by showing good sportsmanship and how I can lift others up along the way. Amen.

I want to love who
I see in the mirror.

Almost every girl, at some point, looks in the mirror and finds something she doesn't like about herself. I went through a phase when I thought my nose was humongous, and I was a bit insecure about it. But humans naturally come in all shapes, sizes, hair colors, skin tones, body types, and so on. And thank God for that! Every girl is unique in her own way, so don't be fooled if society paints a picture that says girls have to look a certain way to be loved. That's wrong! God loves us exactly how we are because He knows that *all* girls are beautiful.

Of course, you should always strive to take care of yourself by eating healthfully, sleeping well, doing physical activities, and practicing good hygiene. But never, *ever* feel like you are inferior because of the way you look. Ultimately, "body shaming" stems from comparisons. If you pick yourself apart and compare your physical appearance to other girls, you risk losing sight of your true beauty. God already validates you in His eyes.

When you establish your identity in Christ, you don't compare yourself to the Instagram model or celebrity magazine cover—both of which, by the way, typically spend *hours* in heavy makeup and styling just to get the final photograph (oh, and then those photos are usually touched up and filtered). So instead of being your own worst critic, look at yourself in the mirror today, knowing that God loves you, and then notice your very best features—a great smile, sincere eyes, strong posture? Do that every day, gorgeous!

The Lord does not look at the things people look at. People look at the outward appearance, but the Lord looks at the heart.

1 Samuel 16:7 NIV

Reflect

Next time you and your girls are hanging out together, make an agreement not to say anything that's self-deprecating—"I hate my toes," or "My artwork stinks." If anyone utters a negative word about herself (or others), call her out to say something positive in its place!

Respond

Get a set of index cards and write down everything you love about yourself. It can be physical features or even internal characteristics like creativity and knowledge. Every day you wake up, repeat at least one card to yourself before you start your day: "I love _____ about myself." Now, use the space here to write a love letter to yourself. Don't hold back!

_____

_____

_____

_____

_____

_____

_____

_____

_____

_____

_____

_____

_____

_____

_____

_____

_____

Jesus, thank you for making me perfectly in your image. It's because of your love that I am able to stand firm in the truth that I am beautifully made. Amen.

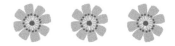

My crush gives me butterflies.

It's possible that there's someone you've been crushing on, or maybe you have a dreamy celebrity crush. And something about that makes you feel all gushy on the inside. It's hard to even explain that feeling you get when your heart seems to leap and your tummy gets all tickly. Crushes are common at around your age, and it's important to know that having a crush is not a sin! Your body is going through many different changes, and your hormones are shifting. This is something that Is completely out of your control. And as your body changes, so do your emotions.

Having feelings for someone is how God created you—you are built for human connection. God wants you to experience happiness and attraction, ultimately through a loving marriage with your spouse. When couples allow God into their union, He guides them so that their bond remains strong. So no matter who your crush is, he should not come before your relationship with God.

What then should you do when you are experiencing overwhelming feelings about a crush? Turn to prayer! God already knows exactly how you feel about your crush, but when you pray and commune with God, you invite Him in to provide divine relationship advice. Plus, it forces you to get your thoughts out of your head so you can process these confusing emotions.

Also consider talking about your feelings with a trusted adult. The Bible says that those who embrace "advice" are accepting wisdom. Be cautious, however, of scrolling on social media for relationship advice. Although you aren't in control of the carnival of crazy hormones in your body, you are totally in charge of what you allow your heart to feel and your eyes to see!

> *You shall love the Lord your God with all your heart, with all your soul, and with all your mind. This is the first and great commandment.*

Matthew 22:37–38 NKJV

Reflect

Although you have a crush, your relationship with God always comes first. So, have you thought about whether your crush cares much about God? The boy is probably adorable beyond words, but how much do you know about his faith?

Respond

Chat with your group of friends about how you can honor God with how you think about your crushes. Use the space provided to create a list of ideal qualities you hope to find in a crush, but here's the catch: Be sure the list does not include *any* physical characteristics.

_____

_____

_____

_____

_____

_____

_____

_____

_____

_____

Jesus, I admit that sometimes I have fuzzy feelings and crushes! I know that it is not a sin to have a crush, but I want to honor you with my feelings. Please give me guidance, wisdom, and courage. Amen.

I can't stop comparing myself to other people.

Did you know that no one else in the entire universe has the same DNA as yours? Even identical twins have qualities that are unique from each other. How cool it is that God created such an amazing mash-up of people? There are superb athletes, studious types, crafty girls, tech geniuses—all kinds of peeps! So why do you sometimes still feel tempted to make comparisons?

Have you noticed that people often want what they don't have? Your curly haired friend wants to straighten her hair, and the friend with stick-straight tresses wishes for curls. Maybe you envy the girl who always gets straight A's while you struggle to maintain a B average. But that same girl trips over her own two feet and is so jealous of your spot on the cheer squad.

Whatever it is that you're comparing yourself to doesn't even stand a chance against what God says about who we are. He wants you to recognize your strengths and uniqueness. He doesn't want you to be a cookie-cutter clone of the girl across the street. He expects you to be uniquely you!

Nothing on this earth compares to the majesty of confidence, hope, and grace embraced through God's love. Apart from Him, you might search for approval by attempting to fit in with "what's trending." But God created you on purpose and for a purpose. He knows every hair on your head and every thought that runs through your mind. He knows that people are different but equal. And He loves you all!

I will praise you because I have been remarkably and wonderfully made. Your works are wonderful, and I know this very well.

Psalm 139:14 HCSB

Reflect

Do you truly believe that God delights in you? Do you believe that God smiles when He thinks of you? He loves *everyone*!

Respond

Psalm 139 is commonly referred to as the Father's Love Letter. Take some time to read this passage and write down everything that God says about you.

_____

_____

_____

_____

_____

Creator, you did not intend for me to compare myself to others. You made me perfectly in your image, and because of that I will stand tall in confidence. Thank you for being a loving Father. Amen.

How can I stay confident?

Confidence is the feeling or belief that you can rely on something. For example, you are probably confident that your math teacher understands math. Confidence can also be how much we believe in ourselves. Are you confident that you are able to graduate high school and even college one day? Do you believe that you are beautiful and strong in the way that God created you? You should be confident in all these things!

Some girls have trouble with self-confidence at your age. If people are saying mean things about you, it can be hard to remember to trust in yourself rather than what people say. Or if you get lost in criticizing yourself, you might tear down your own self-confidence. Don't go there! Always remember that God made you and loves you exactly as you are. God has confidence in you, and you can honor God by having confidence in yourself.

True self-confidence rooted in God is always a good thing! Be mindful, though, that you don't cross over into arrogance. There's a difference between celebrating your hard-earned achievements through the Lord—"I'm so proud of myself for studying hard and doing well on that test"—and being boastful or too arrogant for your own good—"I'm the smartest person in the whole class, so I don't need to study."

Be confident in God's love for you. If you have self-doubts— we all get them!—just think about how God feels about you. God has every confidence in you and knows you can be the best person you can be.

You are my hope, Lord God, my confidence from my youth. I have leaned on you from birth.

Psalm 71:5–6 HCSB

Reflect

Talk to a family member or trusted adult about confidence. Have they ever struggled to have confidence in themselves? (I bet they have!) How did they get through it and remind themselves of God's love?

Respond

Make a list of five ways you can be more confident in yourself, in school, and in your sport if you play one.

1. _____

2. _____

3. _____

4. _____

5. _____

Some days I feel confident but other days I don't feel like I've got it all together. I want to feel confident every day, but I just can't seem to figure it out. I pray that you give me guidance, Jesus!

I feel alone.

Have you ever been up at night, not able to sleep, and it felt like everything was just too much? Ever feel like you don't have anyone close to confide in? Or maybe you're struggling at school ever since your best friend moved away? You might be feeling loneliness. Everyone feels lonely sometimes. Sometimes you might feel alone even in a room full of people—maybe you might feel like you don't belong or like people don't "get you." Or sometimes you might feel lonely when you're dealing with a tough situation—for example, if you're trying to solve a problem on your own.

Yearning to connect with a community or friend group is totally normal! As human beings, we are wired to want to connect with other people. In the Psalms, you can read about how David cried out to God because he felt "lonely and afflicted." David couldn't scroll TikTok or Insta when he felt lonely. Instead, he went directly to the source of all hope and healing: God.

Even though there will be times when you don't get invited to the party or are left out of a group text, remind yourself that you are *never* alone. God will not leave your side. Jesus is nearer than you might ever imagine.

The Lord your God, He is the one who goes with you. He will not leave you nor forsake you.

Deuteronomy 31:6 NKJV

Reflect

Think of times you felt lonely and how you responded. Were you feeling lonely because you felt rejected by someone or left out of the group? Or did you feel all alone in a problem? Maybe you felt alone because you were convinced you couldn't share the problem, or perhaps you felt no one else had ever experienced a similar dilemma.

Respond

Journal in the space provided about lonely feelings you've experienced, and ask God to show you better ways to cope moving forward. Write it as a poem.

_____

_____

_____

_____

_____

I feel really afraid of being alone, God. I start to wonder if anyone cares, and I feel as though no one hears my cries. I believe that you will comfort me in these times of loneliness. I trust you!

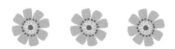

It was just a white lie . . .

Has someone ever lied to you, such as a friend or sibling? It doesn't feel good when you find out that person was lying, does it? When you are honest, it shows that you respect others. If you lie to cover up something you've done, it goes against living an honest life.

Honesty means you are truthful in what you say or do, and it is the bedrock of your character as a believer in Christ. When you are honest with others, it shows that you have integrity and that others can trust you.

People can be dishonest for many reasons. They might be afraid of the consequences, or they don't want to admit that they have fallen short, or maybe they are simply hiding the truth because they are uncomfortable with what's behind the truth. Whatever the case might be, the most important thing to understand is that we are not meant to carry the burden of lying. This is the beautiful grace of God.

The truth about lying is that sometimes people lie with *good* intentions. For instance, maybe your brother told you a big fat lie—he said he didn't break your favorite glass figurine because he didn't want to break your heart. He meant well. He told you it must be misplaced because he thought he could replace it, but then he couldn't find a replica, so he spun a few more lies. And you see, that's what often happens. One lie turns into another lie and another and another, until the whole ordeal is off the rails.

You've heard the old cliché: Honesty is the best policy. That might sound lame, but there's . . . well, *truth* to that saying.

It is better to be poor and honest than to be foolish and tell lies.

Proverbs 19:1 ICB

Reflect

When was the last time you were tempted to tell a lie—even one that seemed really small? What did you choose to do? No matter what decision you made in the past, reflect on how you can avoid the temptation to lie the next time something like this happens.

Respond

Has someone ever lied to you? How did it make you feel? In the space provided, write about what happened and what you learned from it.

_____

_____

_____

_____

Even though it's wrong, sometimes it's easier to tell a white lie instead of telling the truth. Lord, can you help me have the courage to just be honest with others?

I feel creatively blocked.

In the very first verse of the Bible, we learn about one of God's greatest characteristics: His creativity. The ultimate Creator formed the universe, divided the oceans and heavens, gave life to creatures, and brought human life to the earth through Adam and Eve. Obviously, you can't build a universe through your breath, like God did—but you still embody His characteristics. All people were created in His likeness and image, so that means you, too, are creative! You have the ability to do great things in the world, simply by the unique ways you are able to think about topics and bring them to life in different ways.

Creativity is not limited to just artistic or musical abilities, though. Creativity is creating something out of nothing. Just think about it—what other creature on Earth has the ability to conceptualize an idea in their head and put it on paper? Only humans have created clothes, houses, art, music, dance, technology, and so much more . . . all through their creative abilities.

Creativity flows through you, even if you don't realize it. God wants you to embrace your creativity! The Bible says you were created in Christ "to do good works." This means you are meant to use the talents He gave you, to shine His light and love throughout the world. You might not be able to draw. You might not even be able to carry a tune. But there is *something* you can do unlike anyone else in the world! Maybe you're the best-ever babysitter, or you've completely perfected your chocolate chip cookie recipe.

Be encouraged to find the things you are good at and expand on those interests with all your heart! What will you do with your creative talents this week?

In the beginning God created the sky and the Earth.

Genesis 1:1 ICB

Reflect

What unique gifts or talents has God given you? How can you use those to make the world a better place?

Respond

Imagine that you have unlimited resources and materials to build a magnificent masterpiece of some sort. What would you create? Make a rough first-draft drawing of it in the space provided on the next page.

God, thank you for being the ultimate Creator, allowing me to be creative just like you! Would you help me discover my talents and show me how to use them to glorify your name? Amen.

I'm feeling lazy.

Everyone has lazy days when they just feel like they want to sit on the couch and relax. That's an okay, normal feeling to have sometimes, and it's okay to take a day "off" every now and then. But it's also important to regularly power through that feeling and move your body.

Just like you are expected to take care of your room, do well in school, and love your family, you have a responsibility to take care of your body! How are you supposed to go out into the world to do great things if you aren't giving your body what it needs? God gave you the gift of life, so you can show your thankfulness by caring for your body. Exercising can lift your mood, boost your energy, and even help you sleep better. When you move your body, you tend to naturally feel better—and who doesn't want that?

Taking care of yourself through exercise has not only biological benefits, but also psychological and spiritual benefits, as well. The Bible says that "your bodies are temples of the Holy Spirit, who is in you," which is another reason you should love your body.

Feeling lazy? Often it works to just start an activity, even if you feel like you don't want to. Once your body's moving those feelings will usually go away!

Exercising doesn't need to mean you hit the gym like it's boot camp, or you run around the block until you're sweating bullets. It's more about enjoying all the wonderful things your body is able to do—bicycling, roller skating, bowling, volleyball, swimming, hiking—so you can take part in activities you love. If you can get outside to do your exercise, that's wonderful! You're stuck in the house? Blast some music, dance around your bedroom, and give all the glory to God!

Physical exercise has some value, but spiritual exercise is valuable in every way, because it promises life both for the present and for the future.

1 Timothy 4:8 GNT

Reflect

This week, be mindful of how your body feels as you do different activities, like sports and school. How does it feel when you come in from that really intense kickball game at recess? How does it feel in your body, and how does your mood feel? Take a moment and notice how exercise affects your body and mind.

Respond

Make a list here of your favorite fun activities that involve exercise. Draft a schedule for how you might enjoy some of those activities this week.

_____

_____

_____

_____

_____

_____

_____

_____

_____

_____

_____

_____

_____

_____

_____

God, thank you for blessing me with the gift of a
healthy body. I pray for long and joyful lives for
my friends and loved ones. Amen.

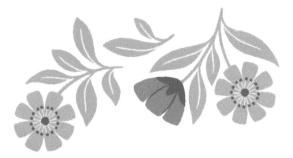

How can I learn from others?

Caregivers and teachers are probably telling you what to do and what not to do, and that can be pretty annoying. You probably feel like you know a lot—and you probably do—but is this confidence rooted in a place of pride where you feel like you *should* know a lot? You might feel mad when someone has to teach you something, but God intended for learning to be a positive experience! Learning from others not only helps you become better at certain things, but it also opens the door to new ideas.

Part of growing up is having others who have gone before you show you the way. That's why learning from others is so great! If someone you look up to explains how they took wrong turns on their journey, you might choose not to make those same mistakes. By learning from others, we avoid having to experience their pain.

When you humble yourself and open your heart to hearing others' stories, you give yourself a chance to experience grace on a whole new level. I can count endless times my mother has given me advice that I actually listened to, and it saved me a lot of heartache and pain. I chose to hear about what she experienced so I wouldn't have to suffer the same way she did.

Ultimately, God wants you to have wisdom. When you listen to and learn from others, you give yourself access to their experiences. You can learn from other people's testimonies and mistakes. And life's lessons aren't just for kids—you will always have access to learning throughout your lifetime!

> *How much better to get wisdom than gold, to get insight rather than silver!*

Proverbs 16:16 NIV

Reflect

Think of someone who has had a positive impact on your life. What did you learn from that person?

Respond

Think of a few people in your life who you look up to and want to learn from, and reach out to them! Write a questionnaire in this space that includes your most pressing Qs about life and God.

_____

_____

_____

_____

> Father, thank you for sending people before me who love me and are wise. Because of your perfect love and grace, I am surrounded by people I can learn from. Thank you, Jesus! Amen.

What will heaven be like?

Imagine a place where everything is perfect and there is no pain, suffering, hatred, fear, or even crying! This is a place where all wrongs are made right, and you are aware that you get to be with Jesus forever. If you're thinking this place sounds like heaven, you're right! Heaven is evidence of God's goodness. He has promised you forever with Him in heaven when your earthly body passes away on Earth.

The beautiful thing about heaven is that as a believer it is your ultimate destination. You will be with God in heaven, where no one suffers. And all you have to do to get to heaven is believe. Believe in what, though? Believe in God! Keep your faith that the Lord made you, loves you, and guides you.

Your perception of heaven is about your own mindset, so your faith is the path to the greatest freedom in this world and beyond. Because of your faith in Jesus, you can talk to the Savior, and nothing you do will ever change His love for you. Take courage in this truth and let this shape how you think about things. You don't have to carry the problems that life throws at you, because you can lay them at the feet of Jesus! Now *that* sounds heavenly.

You have seen how I, the Lord, have spoken to you from heaven.

Exodus 20:22 GNT

Reflect

Have you ever thought about what heaven will be like? What is your vision of heaven on Earth? What actions might you to take to make your world more like heaven?

Respond

Write down the questions you have about heaven. Once you have your list, sit with someone you love and trust and have a conversation about your thoughts.

_____

_____

_____

_____

_____

> If I'm being honest, God, heaven seems really cool, but how can it really exist? When I die will I just go up into the sky? I have so many questions for you, God! Help me to have faith in heaven.

Help me forgive.

Forgiveness can be one of the toughest things you'll have to do in your lifetime, and it is definitely something that takes patience and practice. There might be a time when you need to forgive your sister for accidentally deleting your favorite playlist from your phone, or your little brother because he ruined your favorite pair of jeans by spilling juice on them. Or maybe a friend revealed your most sacred secret to the whole youth group and it really put a dent in your relationship with them.

The truth is that there is always potential for someone to hurt your feelings, and when that happens you have a decision to make. Will you hold a grudge and respond in anger? Or will you take a moment to step back and choose the sometimes-painful option—forgiveness? Forgiveness can get pretty tricky sometimes because it can't be justified in certain situations. Maybe someone intentionally hurt you and you have a reason to be upset with that person. Maybe the person who was supposed to build you up in life was the one who really tore you down, making you feel unseen, rejected, and even hopeless. Hear me, sister, your emotions are validated.

But what happens when we are believers and choose love and peace over pain? When we choose to follow God, we choose forgiveness and are able to release the pain that we are harboring in our hearts. The tricky thing about forgiveness is understanding that most of the time forgiveness is for ourselves and not the other person. Think about it: The person who offended you is not suffering from their actions. YOU are. When we hold on to that pain, it sits in our hearts and holds us back from living in freedom and as God has designed us to live.

Sometimes you'll also have to forgive yourself! Have you ever said that you were going to do something—like study an extra few hours for the big exam, or that you weren't going to gossip negatively—and you fell back on your word? Don't worry, we've all been there. We are not perfect individuals and will fall short in one way or another, which is why we should learn to be gentle and to forgive ourselves. You might even be in a situation where you were the one who hurt someone else and need to ask for forgiveness. It won't always be easy forgiving others, asking others for forgiveness, or forgiving yourself, but one thing will never change, and that's the fact that you are already forgiven and loved by God!

Forgiveness is something that our Father has called us to do for the rest of our lives until we rest in heaven with Him. The most beautiful thing about forgiving others and ourselves is that we have to rely on God for strength. When we rely on the Holy Spirit for the grace to forgive, it is an act of surrendering to God. He sees this as faith, and because of that, He will guide our souls to feel better from the pain that others have caused us.

Be kind and compassionate to one another, forgiving one another, just as God also forgave you in Christ.

Ephesians 4:32 HCSB

Reflect

How has forgiveness changed your life?

Respond

Think of someone you should forgive and ask God to help you release the anger and pain. Journal about your feelings and experience during your quiet time.

_____

_____

_____

_____

_____

Father, I know that at times I can hold on to so much anger and pain. It's hard for me to let go of the pain, but I want to surrender to your will and learn to forgive. Thank you for helping me forgive others! Amen.

I'm struggling with my value.

From music and TV to magazines to your Insta feed, it can feel like everywhere you turn, someone is trying to tell you who to be. With all that noise, it can be hard to remember who you *want* to be—let alone discover who you are. It can feel like an overwhelming amount of pressure to wear the most perfect clothes, have the best-looking body, and show off the coolest hairstyles. Sometimes, what the world says drowns out the voice in your own head and can have you second-guessing some things:

"Am I pretty enough?"

"Does God really love me?"

"Will this outfit make me popular with the kids at school?"

"Am I really whole and free?"

Such questions can sometimes seem to do a total mind takeover. How does this happen? It's the result of defining your worth in worldly stuff. When you believe that what you wear and what you look like defines your worth, you are forgetting that you are already worthy—you have been chosen by your Creator. When you feel small in this world, God says you are more than enough. When you feel forgotten, God reminds you that there is no place you can go where He will not be with you. God says that you are not forsaken, and you are perfectly loved.

The next time you hear negative chatter in your head, remember that the Savior has given you your identity as a child of God. You are who God says you are, so long as you believe.

And that means believing in yourself, too! Walk in the light of truth that you are worthy . . . period.

> *We are God's handiwork, created in Christ Jesus to do good works, which God prepared in advance for us to do.*

Ephesians 2:10 NIV

Reflect

What does scripture say about how God shows that you are worthy in His eyes? Do some Bible research.

Respond

Google-search the song titled "Who You Say I Am" by Hillsong Worship and take some time to *really* listen to the lyrics this week. What verses stand out most to you? Now, write your own song about your self-worth with original lyrics. Sing it out loud!

_____

_____

_____

_____

_____

_____

_____

_____

_____

_____

_____

_____

_____

_____

God, thank you for declaring my identity even
before I was born here on Earth. Will you still my
soul and quiet my mind so I can hear the whisper
of your voice and feel your love? Amen.

God, are you listening?

A lot of times people put prayer in a box that limits it to just closing your eyes and talking to God. But prayer is more than just talking—it's how you communicate with the Lord. Think about how you communicate with your caregivers or friends in lots of different ways, by phone and Internet. Well, you can communicate with God in many ways, too! You can pray through singing, writing, or even stopping to appreciate His creations on your nature walk. God's ear is always tuned toward you. He hears your prayers, sees every tear, and feels every joy you feel because God is all-powerful and is everywhere at all times. Not a second goes by that He is not with you.

Many stories in the Bible share the power of prayer and how God shows up when you need Him: Jesus prays for God's will to be done before his arrest and crucifixion. A synagogue ruler asks Jesus to heal his daughter, so she won't die. Peter prays to be released from prison. Hannah prays desperately to have a baby. In each story, people cry out to God—and he shows up *every* time.

God *always* hears you. When you pray because times are hard, He hears you. When you pray to give thanks for all God has done for you, He hears you. No matter what prompts your prayers, offer them with confidence and faith knowing your almighty Father is able and ready to shower you with answers. Whether you write your prayers, sing them, draw them, or speak them out loud, they do not fall on deaf ears!

Don't worry about anything, but in all your prayers ask God for what you need, always asking Him with a thankful heart.

Philippians 4:6 GNT

Reflect

How can you find more time in your weekly routine to spend time with God in prayer?

Respond

If you normally pray out loud, try journaling your prayers here this week. If you normally journal, pray out loud this week!

_____

_____

_____

_____

_____

I know this is silly, but sometimes praying can feel a little weird because I feel like I'm just talking to myself most of the time. Can you show me that you hear my prayers? God, please help me have faith that you always hear me!

What am I designed to do?

It can be difficult to figure out your life's true purpose. I used to think I was going to be a physical therapist, but I actually ended up being an author and project manager. You can plan your life out to the teensiest detail, but God ultimately knows your best path and will direct you clearly. God says that "before I formed you in your mother's womb," He already had your life planned out. Your story is God's story. Because you have a loving Father, you need not worry about the little details.

Sometimes you aren't going to have it all figured out, and that is okay. You are not meant to carry the burden of being all-knowing, so we should leave that up to our Father in heaven. What then should you do if you're trying to figure out what you want to do with your life in the future? Be encouraged to embrace each moment and experience you encounter in your life *now*. Maybe focus on the classes, sports, or topics you most enjoy and excel at.

It's in those moments—when you discover you have a new passion or learn a new skill—that God speaks to your soul to guide you down your personalized path. Don't beat your brain trying to exactly define your purpose. Take time to explore the things that intrigue you. God gives you little nudges for a reason, and He will guide you!

A man's heart plans his way, but the Lord directs his steps.

Proverbs 16:9 NKJV

Reflect

What do you think you were called to do? Sometimes the people closest to you see things in you that you don't always notice. Sit with a trusted adult and ask what she sees in you as it relates to your purpose in life.

Respond

Use this space to write a paragraph that describes you living your dream job.

_____

_____

_____

_____

_____

_____

> I want to do exactly what it is that you have designed me to do! Father, will you help me understand what that is and how I can achieve it?

I want to make better choices.

Every day, you are faced with decisions that will impact the trajectory of your life. Your daily choices define who you are and how successful you will be in your endeavors. That's why it's important to make smart decisions. No one is perfect, and of course there will be times when you fall short. But most important is where your choices are rooted. Are you being true to yourself and God?

When you know who you are, your decisions come from the solid foundation of God's truth. Think about the choices you are faced with in your day-to-day and how your perspective shapes how you make decisions. The Bible says that humans have free will. That means you have control over the choices you make. That could be something small like what color shirt you pick to wear today—maybe you pick red because it's your favorite color. Or it could be something big, like deciding to tell the truth that it was you who knocked over and broke Mom's vase, because you know telling the truth is the right thing to do. God gives you a choice, because He wants you to choose to follow Him.

What happens when you make a mistake and choose the wrong thing? We've all done that! The amazing thing about God's grace is that no matter what bad decisions you made in the past, you can always make a better decision next time and choose to side with God. Let's say you chose to lie about that vase and say the cat knocked it over. You can't undo that bad choice you made in the past, but you can choose to apologize and come clean to your Mom now. And the next time you're tempted to make a bad decision like lying, you can make a better choice and instead choose to follow the Lord.

In the end, our choices are reflections of what we believe about ourselves and our heavenly Father!

> *If you go the wrong way—to the right or to the left—you will hear a voice behind you. It will say, "This is the right way. You should go this way."*

Isaiah 30:21 ICB

Reflect

What kind of choices have you been making recently and how have they affected others? Have a discussion with your group of friends about how you can commit to making decisions based on faith instead of fear.

Respond

What does the idea of free will mean to you? Do some stream-of-consciousness writing about it in this space. That means you just put pen to paper and scribble out whatever comes to your mind. Don't stop to think about penmanship, punctuation, or spelling!

_____

_____

_____

_____

_____

_____

_____

_____

_____

_____

_____

_____

_____

Jesus, it's hard to make choices, and sometimes
I don't make all of the right decisions. Please help
me figure out the right thing to do, even when
it's confusing!

I need you, God!

Think about a time when you felt like you deserved something. Maybe you did some extra chores around the house to earn allowance money, or maybe you triple-checked your math homework to make sure you'd get that top grade. It's great to work hard for things! But there's one good thing that you can't earn. It's God's grace.

Grace is a gift from God, a demonstration of His kindness and love for His children. But we can't get it by working hard. God gives us His grace completely free! It's unconditional.

What does that mean? God knows we will slip up and make mistakes in our lives. Sometimes really big ones! No one is perfect all the time. But God's grace means that God will always forgive you if you own up to your mistakes and believe that He has forgiven you. He knows you will probably make other mistakes in the future. That's what it means to be human! But God loves you and will forgive you anyway, as long as you trust in Him. It doesn't matter whether you've made one mistake or 100—God will give you grace no matter what.

The Lord's grace is a great example that we can use in our own lives. What does it mean to be gracious to other people? Well, it's sadly true that other people will probably disappoint you sometimes. They are also human and flawed, just like you. But you can channel God's grace and choose to love people regardless of whether they mess up. Will you choose to show others grace like Jesus has shown you grace?

It is by God's grace that you have been saved through faith. It is not the result of your own efforts, but God's gift.

Ephesians 2:8 GNT

Reflect

What are a few ways you can show others grace this week? Carry out at least one kind deed, and do it with poise and a smile!

Respond

Have you ever been given such an amazing gift that you didn't feel like you deserved it or could accept it because it was too much? The gift of grace is awesome, and you *are* deserving of it. Make a drawing here that depicts your vision of God's grace.

I need you to help me understand this whole grace thing. How can I be given such a gift like grace even if you know I will mess up again? Help me understand, God!

My siblings are so stressful!

Not all kids have siblings, but for those who do, it can often be tough to get along with them, especially if there is an age gap. Older siblings are sometimes responsible for looking out for younger siblings, which can be tough. For younger siblings, it can be hard to not feel jealous because older siblings usually get more freedom, like later curfews. Regardless of where you land in the family pecking order, you have a responsibility to treat your siblings with respect and love. There will be disagreement and other times things will be great, but at the end of the day, you are called to treat others how Jesus wants you to!

A story in the Bible describes a rich, young ruler who asked Jesus, "Teacher, what good thing must I do to get eternal life?" Jesus looked at him and advised that he should keep the commandments—one of which was to love your neighbor as you love yourself. Jesus wants you to be selfless and caring toward others, inspiring you to treat others the way you want to be treated. This includes your siblings!

Maybe you have a stepsibling, or you don't have siblings. Being brothers and sisters doesn't just happen through blood! There may be many people in your life, including cousins and friends, who aren't your direct siblings but who are your sisters and brothers in Christ. Sometimes it's hard to get along with someone who isn't your direct sibling ... but that person also might have a different life experience and point of view that helps you look at things differently. Regardless of whether someone is related to you or not, you should always follow God by loving others as you would want to be loved!

> *Whoever claims to love God yet hates a brother or sister is a liar. Whoever does not love their brother and sister, whom they have seen, cannot love God, whom they have not seen.*

1 John 4:20 NIV

Reflect

When you have an interaction with your sibling this week, try to take a different approach by reminding yourself that Jesus wants you to treat them how you would treat yourself. Ask yourself, "What would Jesus do in this situation?"

Respond

In the space provided, write the names of your siblings and stepsiblings. If you don't have any sibs, name your favorite cousin, your best friend who's a guy, and any of your gal pals you would consider to be "like a sister." Now, write a sentence next to each name that pours praise onto that person.

_____

_____

_____

_____

_____

_____

_____

_____

_____

_____

God, even though it can sometimes be challenging to care for my siblings, I know that you see my good deeds and efforts. I pray that you help me with patience and give me strength to better show love toward my siblings! Amen.

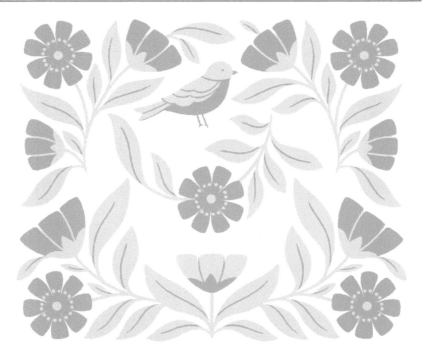

How can I honor God in my relationships?

What does it mean to have a relationship with someone? A relationship doesn't just mean something romantic. You have relationships with most people in your life that you see day-to-day, meaning you have a connection with them that is built over time. It can be hard to navigate all of these relationships!

What does God say about how you should go about this? First, God wants you to honor Him in all that you do, including in your relationships. This means that in your relationships you should resemble God's character. God is love, patience, kindness, and selflessness, and you should strive to honor that in your relationships with others.

In addition to your relationships with friends, family, and classmates, you also have a relationship with yourself. How do you treat your teacher when you disagree with him? How do you treat your little sister when she is upset with you? How do you communicate with your friends if they do something that hurts your feelings? No matter who the person is, you must decide who you want to be in the relationship. Instead of holding grudges, choose forgiveness. Instead of lashing out at someone in a small way, let go of your pride, and communicate how you feel.

Love does not envy; love does not parade itself, is not puffed up; does not behave rudely, does not seek its own, is not provoked, thinks no evil.

1 Corinthians 13:4–7 NKJV

Reflect

When you choose to live by faith, you are choosing to honor God. In your quiet time this week, ask God to show you how you can honor Him in your relationships.

Respond

After you've thought on your own about your relationships, talk to the important people in your life. Over dinner, bring up with your family members what you value about them and how they make you feel. Try to notice the interactions with your friends that make you both feel good!

_____

_____

_____

Relationships can be difficult because sometimes people don't understand me and how I think about things. Will it always be like this, God? I pray that you give me patience in my relationships with others!

What does it mean to be beautiful?

Whether it's the girl in the grade above you who always has perfect hair, or the star you saw on a magazine cover at the grocery store, you might be getting a lot of messages about how you "should" look. Many people think they need to look a certain way in order to be beautiful. This might even seem like you have to wear makeup to be beautiful.

But God created you as you are! In the Lord's eyes, we are all beautiful, because He made us that way. God made you with the face that you have, and God loves who you are. He wants you to embrace the uniqueness that He gave you, both on the inside and outside. The most truly beautiful people give off beauty from the inside, from their character. When you give someone a big smile in the school hallway, or when you reach out your hand to help up a teammate who has tripped—that's beauty.

There's nothing wrong with wanting to look put together, if that's something you want. As you grow up, you might also start to think about wearing makeup. What's important to remember, though, is that God created you as you are. At some point in life, you might want to wear a little bit of makeup to look like yourself on your best day. That's fine! Try chatting with your caregivers about whether that's something you're ready for. Or maybe makeup isn't for you at all. That's fine, too. No matter what you choose, just be sure that you are being true to yourself and the person who God made you to be.

There is only one *you* in this world. You are one of a kind, no matter whether you choose to dress up or not. It's important to remember that you are perfect in God's eyes—you are loved and beautiful. You don't need to prove anything to anyone!

> *What are you doing that you dress yourself in scarlet, that you adorn yourself with gold jewelry, that you enlarge your eyes with paint? You beautify yourself for nothing.*
>
> **Jeremiah 4:30 HCSB**

Reflect

Know that you are loved. Know that you are beautiful. Know that you are perfect in God's eyes. Sit with your friends or maybe even your family and chat about what it means to be beautiful. You'll be amazed at what others believe to be true about beauty!

Respond

Write down a list of attributes you love about yourself, and affirm them every morning this week.

_____

_____

_____

_____

_____

_____

_____

_____

_____

_____

_____

_____

_____

_____

_____

God, thank you for loving me just as I am. Sometimes it can be hard to trust that I'm beautiful because you made me that way. Will you help me embrace my unique beauty?

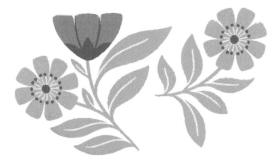

How can I be sure I work hard?

When you were just a little kid, you were probably used to your caregivers telling you what to do and where to go. Now that you're older, it's probably more of your responsibility to make important choices and to make good choices on your own. You know when to use your indoor voice for the classroom and when it's okay to be loud at recess. You know it's up to you to get your homework done and you might not need your caregivers to make sure that happens. All of these things are examples of self-control and discipline.

Scripture describes what's called "the fruit of the spirit," and self-control is one of those fruits. But what are these fruits, and why are they described as spirit? Imagine that you are a fruit tree planted in a large field. You can smell the beautiful flowers all around, you can see water streaming in the meadow, and you feel the sun kissing your tree trunk. Like a tree that is planted and rooted in the ground, you will naturally produce fruit! Now, imagine your favorite fruit growing from all of your tree branches. This is what happens when you are aligned with God. When you are planted firmly in faith and continually shine God's word on your life, you grow in peace, joy, and love—which can be considered fruits on your tree!

But you must do your part to grow those fruits. What does that look like every day? It might be that you get yourself up early so you can help your family prepare breakfast, or you choose to keep doing your homework even when the big finale of your favorite show is on.

We'll never get things right all the time, but we can always choose to try, and to try harder. What will you choose?

The Spirit God gave us does not make us timid, but gives us power, love, and self-discipline.

2 Timothy 1:7 NIV

Reflect

Think about how hard work has helped you meet your goals. What motivated you to put in that discipline? What might have turned out differently if you hadn't worked so hard?

Respond

Think about something you want to become more disciplined in. Journal about it during your quiet time with God this week, and reach out to a trusted loved one who can help you.

_____

_____

_____

> Sometimes I'm tempted to be lazy rather than working hard, and that's just the truth. I know there are times when I should have more self-control. Please help me stay disciplined, God!

It's difficult to stay strong!

Having courage is choosing to do the very things that frighten you. It is about having confidence and boldness when things get tough! Mary, the mother of Jesus, is an amazing example of what it means to embody courage as a woman of God. Mary trusted God, and the way she lived her life showed that faith. When she was told she would give birth to the son of God, she decided to have courage even though it was frightening. She trusted the plan God had for her life!

Another great example of a courageous woman was Queen Esther. Esther was a Jewish woman who asked the king of Persia to spare the Jewish people in his nation by not killing them. During these times, women were not respected and would suffer many consequences if they spoke up directly to a man. But that didn't stop Queen Esther! She trusted in God more than she let fear steer her decisions. She stood firmly with faith and was courageous enough to speak up for her people, saving the Jews. And she likely inspired other women to find their voices as well!

Courage is a choice you will be faced with repeatedly throughout your life. You might need to use your courage if you hear a friend saying something mean about a group of people, and you'll need to have the strength to speak up and say, "That's not okay." When you have deep-rooted faith and know God is behind you, courage surfaces from your heart. Girl, wear God's courage like a superhero cape!

I would have lost heart, unless I had believed that I would see the goodness of the Lord in the land of the living. Wait on the Lord; be of good courage, and He shall strengthen your heart.

Psalm 27:13–14 NKJV

Reflect

How have you been courageous in your past? How did that situation turn out? Ask your family to share with you how they've shown courageousness when things were really hard.

Respond

Write down a list of your fears. In quiet time this week, ask God to show you different ways you can be courageous because of your faith in Him.

_____

_____

_____

_____

> I want to take every opportunity that presents itself to be courageous. In those moments, I pray that you will give me all of the strength to stand tall! Amen.

Who am I, really?

Imagine someone asked you to describe yourself. It's hard, right? And everyone has outside influences, like our caregivers or our classmates, that have an effect on who we feel we should be. We're all so complicated, how do we know who we really are?

Identity is who you are, what you like, your passions, and your purpose—it's about how you perceive yourself. Oftentimes, the world tries to tell you that you are only your past mistakes. It might tell you that because you once cheated on a test, you will always be a cheater. It might tell you that because a parent isnt in your family, that you will always be forgotten. Some people will try to keep you stuck in your past and say that all you'll ever be is the product of the things that hurt you the most.

This is *not* how God sees you! God knows who you are on the inside, and that He created you to be unique. Everyone has their own chalenges, and that's part of the Lord's plan. We all experience ups and downs. Your identity and experiences only belong to you, but we've all been through similar issues. Maybe you and your fiend couldn't be more different—you tried out for field hockey while he auditioned for the community play—but you both know the joy of making the cut!

The more you get to know yourself, the more you can have faith in the person that God created you to be.

God created man in His own image; in the image of God He created him; male and female He created them.

Genesis 1:27 NKJV

Reflect

Think about your life before you decided to have faith in Jesus. What was it like? Now think about your life after you accepted the love of God. How have your viewpoint and identity changed?

Respond

In the space provided, sketch a self-portrait. Break out the colored pencils!

I'm trying to discover who I am, but sometimes I'm torn between who I truly want to be and who I feel like I should be. Will you help me clear these blurred lines, God?

What makes me pure?

When you hear the word "purity," what comes to mind? Purity is meant to describe holiness and cleanliness, and God wants you to embody purity in all aspects of your life.

What probably comes to mind first is purity in relationships. As a believer, you should strive to honor God in your relationships. There might be pressure from friends to live a certain lifestyle, and it might make you feel uncool or weird sometimes for wanting to live purely. When you feel those pressures, trust in God! Know that the Lord has your back and that He is proud of you for sticking with your beliefs. When it comes to your body, know that you should be in control. If anyone tries to make you feel otherwise, talk to a trusted adult.

Purity goes beyond relationships, though! You should try to be pure in your heart and your mind, too. Being pure in your heart and mind means you choose to forgive and let go of past hurts. By not allowing yourself to get clogged up with grudges and other negative emotions, you are in a position to keep it pure before God.

Sometimes, you might make a decision that isn't pure. Everyone makes mistakes, and God knows that we will, because we're human. Guess what? Jesus still loves you! Our God is not hateful. The Lord just wants you to meet Him with who you are now, regardless of what you've done in the past.

Happy are those who are merciful to others; God will be merciful to them! Happy are the pure in heart; they will see God! Happy are those who work for peace; God will call them His children!

Matthew 5:7–9 GNT

Reflect

Sit with your family and talk about what it means to be pure for God. Bring any questions that you have so that you can get the guidance you need.

Respond

Write an affirmation about your commitment to be pure for God. What might you want to say to the Lord about why purity is important to you?

_____

_____

_____

_____

I know that you have called me to live purely for you, Father. Even though there will be times when I fall short, I pray for courage and strength to choose your will over mine. Amen.

How can I give more?

When was the last time you experienced generosity? Maybe a friend shared their cookie with you at lunch, or you gave a toy you'd outgrown to your little sister. Generosity isn't just about items, though. If you explain how to solve a math problem to your classmate, you're being generous with your time.

Generosity was one of the many characteristics Jesus embodied. Jesus always gave to those who had nothing and even those who had everything. He healed sinners, sat with rulers in high places, and visited sick people who were outcast, and He treated them all the same. Jesus was generous with His time and His love, and because of that, you, too, should be generous!

To be generous means to give selflessly. Luke 21:1–3 is a short but beautiful example of what it means to give selflessly. Jesus saw that all of the rich people were putting their gifts into the temple. But he also noticed that a poor widow brought a small gift of two copper coins. Imagine that! This widow had little to nothing, but she still gave what she had from a place of selflessness and faith.

When you put others before yourself and choose to freely give, it's a reflection of what you value. If you value serving others, you will be generous with your time and participate in community service. If you value those who have less than you do, you will donate and give to the underprivileged. All in all, generosity means putting others' needs before your own, and in doing so you honor God.

So how can you be more generous in your community? Maybe you can host a canned food drive at your school to give to the homeless. Maybe being generous looks like writing your teachers a thank-you card as a token of appreciation for all they do. It's important to note here that generosity only has limits that *you* place on it!

> *One person gives freely, yet gains more; another withholds what is right, only to become poor. A generous person will be enriched, and the one who gives a drink of water will receive water.*
>
> **Proverbs 11:24–25 HCSB**

Reflect

How did it make you feel when someone went out of their way to be generous toward you? Think about that and about how it would feel to "pay it forward." Try brainstorming with your family a way you can all be generous. Maybe there's a local food bank or another way you can help people in your community!

Respond

Make a top-ten list of ways you can be generous this week, and challenge your friends and family to join you!

_____

_____

_____

_____

_____

_____

_____

_____

_____

_____

_____

_____

_____

_____

_____

_____

Giving back to others is the right thing to do and I want to do just that. I want to be the most generous, like you! Lord, can you help me remember to be generous?

My friends are influencing me.

Think about the moment you sit down at the lunch table every day at school. What are your feelings? If you feel like the friends sitting with you have your back, awesome! But if you feel a tickle in your stomach, you might want to reflect further on why you could feel that way.

Sometimes classmates or friends, whether they realize it or not, might influence how you feel about yourself and the choices you make. When it seems like everyone is wearing the same thing, or listening to the same music, it can be hard if what your friends like isn't what speaks to you. Instead, trust your gut! That's how the Lord is sharing His plan.

Scripture tells you that as a believer you are "set apart as holy." What exactly does that mean? When someone chooses to accept the love of Christ in her life and is saved by grace through faith, she is given a new identity. God no longer sees her past mistakes. She becomes brand-new.

It's really hard, but even if friends are making different choices, we can still choose to honor the Lord. When friends are in your face, pressuring you to do something that's way outside your comfort zone, who will you be?

Does this sound as if I am trying to win human approval? No indeed! What I want is God's approval! Am I trying to be popular with people? If I were still trying to do so, I would not be a servant of Christ.

Galatians 1:10 GNT

Reflect

Ask God to show you how you can be a light for His glory! Pray, too, for guidance on how you might be able to positively influence the kids who like to pressure their peers.

Respond

Write down a few snappy comebacks that you can use in the face of peer pressure.

_____

_____

_____

_____

_____

_____

_____

_____

_____

_____

_____

_____

_____

_____

_____

_____

Jesus, thank you for being such a loving Father that you give us strength when we are weak. Sometimes fighting peer pressure is hard, because I worry that people will think I'm not cool, but I choose to walk in your truth instead! Amen.

Help me be strong!

Would you believe me if I told you that nothing happens by accident? Everything that has happened in your life was on purpose and for the purpose of making you a stronger young woman. Every tear you've cried, every argument you've gotten into with your siblings or friends, and every difficult situation you've gone through was to make you stronger! Even though those trials might have hurt, the beautiful thing is that you learned something from the situation.

But what happens when you've met your wit's end and you feel like you can't find any more strength? What happens when you get to a time where you've lost all hope and don't know what to do or where to go? This is where learning to find your strength in God comes to life. Scripture tells us that those who struggle will be blessed, and that those who weep and mourn will find joy. How can these opposites happen? Because they are rooted in the Spirit of God and not our own strength.

When things get tough, be encouraged to do these three things: First, honor the emotions that you are feeling. If you are angry, feel the anger. If you are hurting, feel the hurt. Don't ignore the emotions and suppress them. Second, remind yourself that even though you feel these difficult emotions, you can rely on God's strength to get you through. Try to shift your perspective from the issue you are facing to Jesus instead. Finally, speak life over your situation. What does scripture say about having and finding strength in Jesus? Speak those verses over your life and watch your situation shift for the better!

*People who trust the Lord will become strong
again. They will be able to rise up as an eagle in
the sky. They will run without needing rest. They
will walk without becoming tired.*

Isaiah 40:31 ICB

Reflect

When you are weak, you can find strength in Jesus! But how?
Well, first things first: You have to ask Him for strength! Jesus will
meet you right where you are—in the hurt, pain, and mess!—
and all it takes is you acknowledging your need for Him. Then, let
Him do the rest!

Respond

Take time this week to find four verses about strength in Jesus.
Keep them handy for when times get difficult!

1. _____

2. _____

3. _____

4. _____

How can I rely on you for strength when you are
not standing right next to me, God? I want to be
strong but sometimes I don't feel like I can do it.
Will you help make it make sense?

Help me work harder!

Up until now in your life I'm sure you have heard people tell you to do your best and give your all in everything that you do. I'm also pretty sure that the reason they are telling you to work hard is so that you will become successful and all of your dreams will come true.

In Luke 18, Jesus shared a short story to illustrate the bigger picture of what it looks like to persevere. In this parable that he shared with the disciples, he told the story of a woman who requested that a judge—who did not believe in God—"grant her justice against her adversary." She wanted justice to be shown to those who wronged her, but he steadily refused. Daily, this woman continued to ask the judge to grant her justice, and I bet you can guess what happened. Because of her persistence and perseverance, the judge *finally* honored her request!

While it is true that if you work hard and are disciplined you can achieve what you put your mind to—much like the strong woman in the parable—I'd like to offer you a different perspective. Sometimes we get so caught up in the work that we do in the world that we find our worth in it. If you don't get straight A's, you might feel like you are not smart. If you don't perform well in whatever sport you play, you might feel worthless and not valuable to your team. What if you decide to take the value of the work that you do and place it at the feet of Jesus? What if you work hard because you want to honor God with the talents He has given you? This is what it means to glorify God by working hard and giving your all in everything that you do.

The next time that you feel pressure to work hard because of external factors, take a moment to step back and realize who your heavenly Father is and what He says about you. Jesus says that you are loved, whole, perfect, redeemed, and worthy. Let that be the motivating factor for why you work hard!

We must not become tired of doing good. We will receive our harvest of eternal life at the right time. We must not give up!

Galatians 6:9 ICB

Reflect

Spend some time this week in prayer asking God to reveal to you what your true motivations in life are. Ask Him to help you lay those at His feet so that you can replace them with what He says is true about you.

Respond

Write a letter to your future self. Imagine yourself working hard for something but needing help staying in a faithful mindset for the long haul. What would you say to her to help her keep faith?

_____

_____

_____

_____

_____

_____

_____

_____

_____

_____

_____

_____

I get tired, God, and sometimes I don't feel like
I have the strength to do what I said I was going to
do. I want to work hard but I need you to help me
get through it!

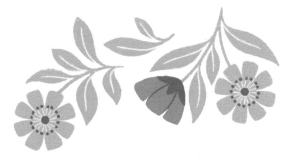

How can I deal with loss?

When we lose something or someone we love, it can be such a hard thing to process. Ever felt sad, angry, hopeless, or upset because you lost someone? Those are all emotions that are associated with the process of grief. Grieving a loss is never easy and I am not here to tell you that it will ever get easier, but as believers, we have a different narrative. When we are suffering, we can have peace because of Jesus. When we are confused, we can have peace of mind. When we are struggling to breathe because the weight of grief is suffocating us, our Father in heaven can breathe new life into us. You are NEVER alone. Jesus is always near and He sees, hears, and feels the pain that you feel.

Be encouraged that when you are grieving there is hope available to you. There is a silver lining in the dark cloud and that is faith and hope in Jesus. When the soldiers moved the stone from the tomb that Jesus was buried in to see that he indeed was not there, that was *proof* that life is everlasting because of Jesus's resurrection! If Jesus had not risen from the grave, we also would not have the gift of life forever in heaven with God.

When you feel grief, don't suppress the feeling, but embrace the pain you feel. Might sound confusing, right? The reality is that when you feel the overwhelming pain from grief but choose to seek God, you will find stillness! If a loved one has passed away and it seems like there is no light at the end of the tunnel, rest assured that they are in the hands of God! Lean into the emotions you feel, and trust and believe that God will meet you right in the pain. He is telling you not to give up and to lean on your support group around you!

He heals the brokenhearted. He bandages their wounds. He counts the stars and names each one. Our Lord is great and very powerful. There is no limit to what He knows.

Psalm 147:3–5 ICB

Reflect

Sit with someone you trust—your caregivers, a mentor, or a friend—and be honest about what you are grieving. Ask them to pray with you so that you can find strength and peace in Jesus.

Respond

What are some things that you are grieving right now? How can you lay them at the feet of Jesus? Write your thoughts down here.

_____

_____

_____

I know that you say I can have peace when I am grieving, but I just don't understand that. Please, Jesus, can you comfort me when I've lost something that means so much to me?

What does it mean to love learning?

————

The majority of our lives until adulthood are spent in three places: home, school, and our communities. Maybe you're a part of a youth group that meets weekly or monthly, so you spend a lot of time with that group of people in your church. Some of those same girls might even go to the same school as you—the place you spend the second-most time. And of course your home—the place where you eat, sleep, and have dance parties while you're getting ready for youth group or school.

While you might enjoy one place more than another, school has gathered potential to change your life even if it might not seem like it at the moment. Although school is very structured with long hours and sometimes difficult subjects to master, there is no way around it. We all have to go through elementary, middle, and high school, and if you desire to further your education you'll go through college! Simply put, there is no way around school except through it.

I'd like to challenge you to shift your perspective on school, though. Instead of thinking about school as a place you have to go because you are required to, try thinking about it as an opportunity to learn something new so that you can grow in wisdom. As believers we are called to give our all to everything that we do, and that includes school! I want to challenge you even more to adopt a different outlook by taking on the perspective that school is your community. Instead of just going to class and doing extracurricular activities, how can you be a light for others? How can you glorify God through your positive influence on others? No matter what your current situation is with school, you have an opportunity to change someone's life by how you choose to honor God through school.

> *I will make your pinnacles of rubies, your gates of crystal, and all your walls of precious stones. All your children* shall *be taught by the Lord, and great* shall *be the peace of your children.*

Isaiah 54:12–13 NKJV

Reflect

How can you change your perspective on school through the lens of community?

Respond

Ask a teacher you trust to help you brainstorm how you can be a positive influence for your peers in school! Write down what you learned here.

_____

_____

_____

_____

_____

_____

_____

_____

_____

_____

_____

_____

_____

God, if I am being honest, sometimes I don't like school. Because you are the light of my life, I am choosing to shift my perspective to view school as an open door for change within my community. Please guide me and show me how to shine for your glory. Amen.

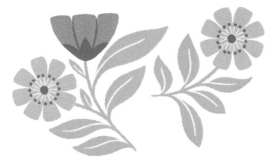

Should I do it? I feel so tempted!

When you think of temptation, what comes to mind? Does it make you think about telling a little white lie to your parents so that you don't get in trouble? Does it make you think about sneaking that $5 from your mother's purse? Maybe temptation makes you think about choosing not to study for an exam. No matter what comes to mind, temptation is something that you will encounter for the rest of your life.

Although God wants his children to live holy and pure lives, the enemy has the total opposite in mind. The evil one's main goal is to steal, kill, and destroy. He wants to steal our joy and hope, kill our confidence, and destroy our faith. This is why we must do our best to avoid and resist temptation.

So how can you fight temptation? If you look at Jesus's life you can see that he, too, had many encounters with temptation. Specifically, He was fasting in the wilderness for 40 days, and that is where the enemy tried to derail Him from what God had called Him to do. The way Jesus combatted temptation was by speaking the word of God over every temptation presented. With the strength of the Holy Spirit, we, too, can resist temptation through prayer and the word of God. When you are in the face of adversity and have to make a decision, ask yourself this: "What does the word of God say about this?" Another great way to fight the struggles of temptation is through accountability to your community. Share with your close friends and family the things you might be struggling with, and ask them to pray for you and to help you stay accountable. It's important to note that you can also put yourself in a position to avoid temptation by making and staying dedicated to strong habits for yourself. This can look like you studying in a dedicated area without distractions, or even choosing not to hang out with a friend in order to get your studying done.

All in all, temptation will not waver, but as your faith grows you will get stronger through every trial and tribulation.

> *No temptation has overtaken you except what is common to humanity. God is faithful, and He will not allow you to be tempted beyond what you are able, but with the temptation He will also provide a way of escape so that you are able to bear it.*

1 Corinthians 10:13 HCSB

Reflect

How can you do a better job of not putting yourself in a position to be tempted?

Respond

Pray and ask God how you can learn to find strength in Him when you are tempted. Journal your thoughts here during quiet time this week.

_____

_____

_____

_____

_____

_____

_____

_____

_____

_____

It's so hard to say no when I am tempted (especially if it's my favorite candy). Why do we always have to resist temptations? Help me, Lord, to stay strong when I'm tempted.

How can I get along better with my family?

Not all families are the same. Maybe you have siblings, or maybe you don't. Maybe you have stepsiblings. Your caregivers could include parents, stepparents, grandparents, other relatives, or foster parents. You could come from a big family with lots of cousins and aunts and uncles, or yours might be a small family. You might even have a family pet. But no matter who is in your family, God gave you those people to love you, care for you, and guide you as you grow up. Love is what makes a family a family.

The truth is, no matter who is in your family, family life can get messy sometimes! We don't get to choose who our families are but we do get to choose how we treat them. Your family will always be one of the voices of influence in your life, especially as you grow and mature as a woman. Now you might be thinking that your siblings can be annoying or maybe your caregiver upsets you sometimes. This is all normal and a part of the good and bad that comes with family life. No matter what, it's important to remember that family is all we have on this side of heaven.

Scripture tells us that we should honor our mothers and fathers. This means that you should show your caregiver the utmost respect no matter what. Ultimately, God has gifted us with caregivers to help guide us through the world, to protect us, and provide for us as we transition into adulthood. Showing respect and love to not only our caregivers but all of our extended family is the ultimate action of love, which is what Jesus desires from us all!

So how can you honor family? Be encouraged to put your phone away when there is scheduled family time so that the time spent together is high quality! We all know what it feels like to have a conversation with someone who is physically present but mentally not paying attention. Maybe honoring your family means that you actually take the initiative to reach out to your loved ones and ask them how they are doing. All in all, when we honor our families, we are honoring God!

Anyone who does not provide for their relatives, and especially for their own household, has denied the faith and is worse than an unbeliever.

1 Timothy 5:8 NIV

Reflect

This week, ask God to show you how you can be a better daughter, sibling, and friend for those you love.

Respond

What do you love most about your family? Make a list of your favorite qualities in your family. You can include all the fun ways you like to spend time together, too!

_____

_____

_____

_____

_____

_____

_____

_____

_____

_____

_____

_____

Jesus, thank you for not letting us do life alone.
Thank you for friends and family and for the
unconditional love that we share. I pray that
you continue to bless us and cover us in Jesus's
name. Amen.

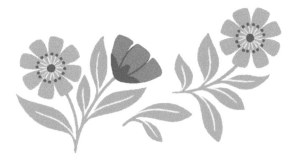

Friends are forever!

In your lifetime you will meet tons of people, some of whom will become the greatest friends you will ever have! There is no better feeling than knowing you can always have your best friend or girlfriend to call when you need a shoulder to lean on. As humans, we are wired for connection and need healthy relationships to thrive in the world. We were not meant to walk this journey of life alone!

Think about the 12 disciples who traveled with Jesus throughout His ministry. Imagine what it would be like to spend nearly every single day with the friends closest to you. Can you imagine how they encouraged one another when times were hard? How they cried together, laughed together, loved people together, and loved Jesus together? True friends are meant to do life with us.

It's important that we choose good friends who have a positive influence on us. Just like the 12 disciples had things in common and were striving for the same things in life, we need a similar community. A good friend is one who supports you, encourages you, and even kindly corrects you when you are wrong. Good friends are those who want the best for you and are selfless. Everyone is different and has unique aspirations, but it's important to have a group of people who support one another, love one another, and correct one another with love to maintain accountability. Friends are everything!

Some friendships do not last, but some friends are more loyal than brothers.

Proverbs 18:24 GNT

Reflect

Have you made any bad choices when picking friends? How can you choose better friends?

Respond

Gather your group of friends and share with one another what you love about your friendships! Write what you learned in the space provided.

_____

_____

_____

_____

_____

My friends mean the world to me! I pray that you continue to bless us and help us be supportive—even if we get upset with one another! Amen.

About the Author

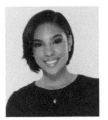 **Jaseña S'vani** was born and raised in Atlanta, Georgia, where she grew up as a pastor's kid and avid athlete. At Georgia State University, she studied exercise science and cheered competitively! After attending The Ultimate Training Camp for Christian student athletes, Jaseña gave her life to Christ and started her walk with Jesus.

Jaseña is passionate about living a life to serve others through sharing her story in writing and art. She hopes that the gifts that God has granted her shine a new light for young people around the world. She wants her life to be a demonstration of what it means to live a life worthy of your individual purpose by utilizing your God-given gifts.